# CONTENTS

# INTRODUCTION

Do you feel like making a significant lifestyle change? Are you willing to improve your life and to start looking and feeling awesome?

Then you are probably in the best place!

We are about to show you that you can become a new person in no time just by making some small but very important changes!

So, here we go!

The first change you need to make regards your dietary habits! Therefore, you need to forget about the meals you are used to eating! You need to focus on adopting a new diet and we think that the best one for you would be the vegan one!

Don't be afraid! This diet might seem to be pretty hard to follow but in fact, it's rather simple!

Veganism just means you have to exclude the consumption of all kind of animal products. You will have to exclude dairy products, eggs, honey and meat.

Instead, you get to eat a lot of veggies, legumes, grains and fruits.

This brings us to the second change you need to make in order to look and feel great! It's the way you cook your meals!

You need to forget about greasy meals, about fat ingredients!

If you decided to become a vegan, you should probably find a healthier way to cook your dishes!

We want to help you with this aspect as well and that's why we suggest you to try using an air fryer instead of your regular pans and pots.

Air fryers cook your meals using rapid air technology. This means that you can cook, steam, bake everything in such a healthy way!

You don't need to use a lot of oil or fat because you can count on the circulation of hot air to cook your meals!

So, what do you say? Are you willing to give veganism a chance?

And if that's the case, are you willing to try cooking your vegan dishes in your amazing air fryer?

If the answer is "yes", then you should know you've made the best decision!

# Appetizers And Snack Recipes

### 1.  Eggplant Appetizer Salad

Servings: 4
Cooking Time: 20 Minutes
**Ingredients:**
- 1½ cups tomatoes, chopped
- 3 cups eggplant, cubed
- 6 ounces black olives, pitted and sliced
- 2 teaspoons balsamic vinegar
- 1 tablespoon oregano, chopped
- Salt and black pepper to the taste

**Directions:**
1. In a pan that fits your Air Fryer, mix tomatoes with eggplant, olives, vinegar, oregano, salt and pepper, toss, introduce in your fryer and cook at 370 ° F for 20 minutes.
2. Divide between small appetizer plates and serve as an appetizer.

### 2.  Easy Zucchini Chips

Servings: 6
Cooking Time: 30 Minutes
**Ingredients:**
- 3 zucchinis, thinly sliced
- Salt and black pepper to the taste
- 2 tablespoons olive oil
- 2 tablespoons balsamic vinegar

**Directions:**
1. In a bowl, mix oil with vinegar, salt and pepper and whisk well.
2. Add zucchini slices, toss to coat well, introduce in your air fryer and cook at 350 degrees F for 30 minutes.
3. Divide zucchini chips into bowls and serve them cold as a snack.
4. Enjoy!

### 3.  Tandoori Chickpeas

Servings: 4
Cooking Time: 10 Minutes
**Ingredients:**
- 3/4 teaspoon of salt
- 19 ounces can of chickpeas (drain and rinse)
- 2 teaspoons of masala or any other spice blend of your choice
- 1 tablespoon of olive oil

**Directions:**
1. Preheat the air fryer to a temperature of 390 degrees Fahrenheit.

2. Get a large-sized bowl and pour in the olive oil and chickpeas. Sprinkle with salt and spices and toss to mix.
3. Eject the fry basket of the air fryer and arrange the chickpeas in a single layer on it. Reinsert the air fryer basket and set the timer to cook for eight to ten minutes. Shake the chickpeas halfway through the timer count. Once the timer elapses, take out the chickpeas and allow to sit and cool on a baking sheet. Repeat the process for leftover chickpeas (a can of chickpeas can take two batches).

### 4.  Cheesy Potato Wedges

Servings: 4
Cooking Time: 16 minutes
**Ingredients:**
- To make the potatoes:
- 1/2 teaspoon of garlic powder
- 1 pound of fingerling potatoes
- 1 teaspoon of kosher salt
- 1 teaspoon of olive oil (extra virgin variety)
- 1 teaspoon of black pepper (ground)
- To prepare the cheese sauce:
- 2 tbsp to 1/4 cup of water
- 2 tablespoons of nutritional yeast
- 1/2 cup of raw cashews
- 1/2 teaspoon of paprika
- 1 teaspoon of fresh lemon juice
- 1/2 teaspoon of turmeric (ground)

**Directions:**
1. Start by preheating the air fryer for three minutes at a temperature of 400 degrees Fahrenheit. Wash and cut the potatoes into halves lengthwise. Rinse and put them into a large-sized bowl. Sprinkle with garlic powder, pepper, salt, and oil and toss to coat thoroughly. Move the potatoes into the air fryer's basket and cook for about 16 minutes. Stop the air fryer seven to eight minutes into the cooking and shake the basket.
2. Get a blender (high-speed variety) and mix the lemon juice, nutritional yeast, paprika, turmeric, and cashews. Begin blending at slow speed, and gradually increase the speed, adding water when necessary. Take care to avoid using

excess water, as the ingredients are required to have a thick and cheesy consistency.
3. Move the cooked potatoes onto a piece of parchment paper or into the air fryer-safe pan. Drizzle the potato wedges with cheese sauce. Return the pan into the air fryer and set the timer and temperature to run for two minutes and 400 degrees Fahrenheit respectively.

### 5.    Basil Crackers

Servings: 6
Cooking Time: 17 Minutes
**Ingredients:**
- ½ teaspoon baking powder
- Salt and black pepper to the taste
- 1 and ¼ cups whole wheat flour
- ¼ teaspoon basil, dried
- 1 garlic clove, minced
- 2 tablespoons vegan basil pesto
- 2 tablespoons olive oil

**Directions:**
1. In a bowl, mix flour with salt, pepper, baking powder, garlic, cayenne, basil, pesto and oil, stir until you obtain a dough, spread this on a lined baking sheet that fits your air fryer, introduce in the fryer at 325 degrees F and bake for 17 minutes.
2. Leave aside to cool down, cut crackers and serve them as a snack.
3. Enjoy!

### 6.    Cinnamon Mango Dip

Servings: 4
Cooking Time: 20 Minutes
**Ingredients:**
- 1 shallot, chopped
- 1 tablespoon vegetable oil
- ¼ teaspoon cardamom powder
- 2 tablespoons ginger, minced
- ½ teaspoon cinnamon powder
- 2 mangos, peeled and chopped
- 2 red hot chilies, chopped
- 1 apple, cored and chopped
- 1 and ¼ cup stevia
- 1 and ¼ apple cider vinegar

**Directions:**
1. In a pan that fits your air fryer, combine shallot with oil, cardamom, ginger, cinnamon, mangos, chilies, apple, stevia and vinegar, stir, introduce in the fryer and cook at 365 degrees F for 20 minutes.
2. Stir the dip really well, divide into bowls and serve.
3. Enjoy!

### 7.    Potato Rosemary Chips

Servings: 4
Cooking Time: 30 Minutes
**Ingredients:**
- 4 potatoes, scrubbed, peeled and cut into thin strips
- A pinch of sea salt
- 1 tablespoon olive oil
- 2 teaspoons rosemary, chopped

**Directions:**
1. In a bowl, mix Potato Rosemary Chips with salt and oil, toss to coat, place them in your air fryer's basket and cook at 330 degrees F for 30 minutes.
2. Divide them into bowls, sprinkle rosemary all over and serve as a snack.
3. Enjoy!

### 8.    Chickpeas With Cumin Snack

Servings: 4
Cooking Time: 20 Minutes
**Ingredients:**
- 15 ounces canned chickpeas, drained
- ½ teaspoon cumin, ground
- 1 tablespoon olive oil
- 1 teaspoon smoked paprika
- Salt and black pepper to the taste

**Directions:**
1. In a bowl, mix chickpeas with oil, cumin, paprika, salt and pepper, toss to coat, place them in the fryer's basket, cook at 390 degrees F for 10 minutes and transfer to a bowl.
2. Serve as a snack
3. Enjoy!

### 9.    Jicama Fries

Servings: 4
Cooking Time: 15 Minutes
**Ingredients:**
- Pepper and salt
- 1 tsp of paprika (smoked variety)
- 1 medium-sized jicama (chop into matchsticks)

- 2 tbsp of olive oil
- ½ tsp of garlic powder

**Directions:**
1. Get a large-sized bowl and pour in the olive oil, jicama matchsticks, and smoked paprika. Sprinkle with pepper, salt and garlic powder.
2. Toss the ingredients to combine well until every jicama matchstick is properly coated in spices and oil.
3. Set the timer and temperature of the air fryer to 15 minutes and 400 degrees Fahrenheit respectively. After four or five minutes, shake the basket to ensure the jicama matchsticks get mixed evenly.
4. Best served hot with ketchup as dip or any other condiment of your choice.

### 10. Oil-free Potato Chips With Garlic Parm Flavor

Servings: 4
Cooking Time:30 minutes.
**Ingredients:**
- 2 tablespoons of vegan parmesan (homemade)
- 2 teaspoons of salt
- 2 large-sized potatoes (red variety)
- 4 cloves of garlic (minced or crushed)

**Directions:**
1. Slice the red potatoes thinly. It is advised to use a mandolin knife with a 5 millimeter blade.
2. Get a bowl and put the potato slices in. Fill the bowl with water. Sprinkle with two teaspoons of salt and allow to sit and soak for 30 minutes.
3. Drain the potatoes and rinse in running water. Pat dry with paper towels.
4. Pour the vegan parmesan and minced garlic with the potatoes and toss to mix.
5. Make a layer in the air fryer using slices of potatoes, in no more than 4 layers or thereabouts. Ensure to not overload the air fryer so that the chips can cook evenly.
6. Set the temperature to 179 degrees Fahrenheit and the timer to 20 to 25 minutes. Fry until the potatoes become dry and lose their flimsiness. Toss and stir the basket every five minutes.
7. Increase the temperature to about 400 degrees and proceed to let the potatoes

sit for another five minutes or until the potatoes reach a state of crunchiness.
8. Take out the potatoes from the air fryer and spread with salt and more vegan parmesan.
9. Repeat the same process for the remaining halves of the sliced potatoes.
10. Your snack is ready to serve.

### 11. Mini Peppers Appetizer

Servings: 6
Cooking Time: 6 Minutes
**Ingredients:**
- 1 pound mini bell peppers, halved
- Salt and black pepper to the taste
- 1 teaspoon garlic powder
- 1 teaspoon sweet paprika
- ½ teaspoon oregano, dried
- ¼ teaspoon red pepper flakes
- 2 cups soft tofu, crumbled
- 1 tablespoons chili powder
- 1 teaspoon cumin, ground

**Directions:**
1. In a bowl, mix chili powder with paprika, salt, pepper, cumin, oregano, pepper flakes, tofu and garlic powder and stir.
2. Stuff pepper halves with this mix, place them in your air fryer's basket and cook them at 350 degrees F for 6 minutes.
3. Arrange peppers on a platter and serve them as an appetizer.
4. Enjoy!

### 12. Squash Party Muffins

Servings: 6
Cooking Time: 26 Minutes
**Ingredients:**
- 1 spaghetti squash, peeled and halved
- 2 tablespoons avocado mayonnaise
- 1 cup cashew cheese, shredded
- 1 and ½ cups vegan breadcrumbs
- 1 teaspoon parsley, dried
- 1 garlic clove, minced
- Salt and black pepper to the taste
- Cooking spray

**Directions:**
1. Put squash halves in your air fryer, cook at 350 degrees F for 16 minutes, leave aside to cool down, scrape flesh into a bowl, add salt, pepper, parsley, breadcrumbs, mayo and cashew cheese and stir well.

2. Spray a muffin tray that fits your air fryer with cooking spray and divide squash mix in each cup, introduce in the fryer and cook at 360 degrees F for 10 minutes.
3. Arrange muffins on a platter and serve as a snack.
4. Enjoy!

### 13. Crispy Fried Pickles

Servings:4
Cooking Time:20 Minutes
**Ingredients:**
- 14 thickly cut dill pickle slices (Crunchy refrigerated pickles are best.*)
- ¼ cup all purpose flour
- ⅛ teaspoon baking powder
- 3 Tablespoons dark beer (All German beer is vegan.)
- Pinch of salt
- 2 to 3 Tablespoons water
- 2 Tablespoons cornstarch
- 6 Tablespoons panko bread crumbs
- ½ teaspoon paprika
- Pinch of cayenne pepper
- Oil spray (for air frying) or organic canola oil (for frying in skillet)
- ¼ to ½ cup vegan ranch dressing (Follow Your Heart ranch is my favorite.)

**Directions:**
1. Dry the pickle slices on a clean kitchen towel, making sure to dry each side. Set aside.
2. In a small bowl, combine all purpose flour, baking powder, dark beer, pinch of salt, and 2 Tablespoons of water. The batter should be thick but pourable, like waffle batter. If it›s too thick, add an additional Tablespoon of water. Set the beer batter aside.
3. Put out two dinner plates. On one plate, sprinkle cornstarch. On the second plate, combine panko bread crumbs, paprika, cayenne pepper, and another pinch of salt.
4. Now it›s time to bread the pickles. Make an assembly line on your counter with pickles, then cornstarch, then beer batter, and then panko mixture. If you›re air frying, put the air fryer basket at the end of the assembly line.

If you›re frying them, put an additional plate for battered pickles.
5. One pickle at a time, put the pickle slice in cornstarch on each side. Tap to remove excess cornstarch. This will make it easier for the batter to stick to the slice. Then dip the slice in beer batter, making sure to evenly coat it. Allow the slice to drip off any excess batter before continuing to the panko. Dredge the slice in the panko mixture, fully covering it.
6. If air frying: Put the slice into the air fryer. Continue with all of the dill pickle slices, making sure that they are in a single even layer in the air fryer basket. Give a spritz with spray oil. Air fry for 8 minutes at 360 degrees, stopping once halfway through to flip all of the slices and give another spritz of oil. After 8 minutes, check that they are the desired amount of toasty brown. If needed, air fry for an additional minute.
7. If frying in skillet: Continue battering all of the dill pickle slices, and put each breaded slice on the final plate. Cover the skillet in a thin layer of organic canola oil. Bring to a medium high heat. Test the oil is hot enough by dropping a few panko crumbs into the oil. If the oil immediately bubbles around it, it›s ready to go. Put the breaded dill pickle slices into the oil. Depending on the size of your skillet, you may need to work in batches. You don›t want to overcrowd, or else they won›t brown properly. Fry for 3 minutes on one side, flip all of the pickle slices, and fry for an additional 1 to 2 minutes, until they are toasty brown. Move to a towel-covered plate to drain.
8. Serve with vegan ranch dressing.

### 14. Sesame Chard Spread

Servings: 4
Cooking Time: 7 Minutes
**Ingredients:**
- 2 garlic cloves, minced
- 2 cup chard leaves
- ½ cup veggie stock
- ¼ cup sesame paste
- Salt and black pepper to the taste
- A drizzle of olive oil

- Juice of 1 lemon

**Directions:**
1. In a pan that fits your air fryer, mix stock with chard, salt and pepper, stir, introduce in the fryer and cook at 320 degrees F for 7 minutes.
2. Drain chard, transfer to your food processor, add garlic, sesame paste, lemon juice, olive oil and parsley, pulse well and divide into bowls and serve.
3. Enjoy!

### 15. Tofu Snack

Servings: 4
Cooking Time: 20 Minutes
**Ingredients:**
- 12 ounces firm tofu, cubed
- 1 teaspoon sweet paprika
- 1 teaspoon sesame oil
- 1 tablespoon coriander, chopped
- 2 tablespoons coconut aminos

**Directions:**
1. In a bowl, mix paprika with the oil, coriander and aminos, whisk well, add tofu pieces, toss to coat and leave aside for 30 minutes.
2. Transfer tofu cubes to your air fryer's basket and cook at 350 degrees F for 20 minutes shaking halfway.
3. Transfer them to a bowl and serve as a snack.
4. Enjoy!

### 16. Cauliflower Crackers With Italian Seasoning

Servings: 12
Cooking Time: 25 Minutes
**Ingredients:**
- 1 big cauliflower head, florets separated and riced
- ½ cup cashew cheese, shredded
- 1 tablespoon flax meal mixed with 1 tablespoon water
- 1 teaspoon Italian seasoning
- Salt and black pepper to the taste

**Directions:**
1. Spread cauliflower rice on a lined baking sheet that fits your air fryer, introduce in the fryer and cook at 360 degrees F for 10 minutes.
2. Transfer cauliflower to a bowl, add salt, pepper, cashew cheese, flax meal and Italian seasoning, stir really well, spread this into a rectangle pan that fits your air fryer, press well, introduce in the fryer and cook at 360 degrees F for 15 minutes more.
3. Cut into medium crackers and serve as a snack.
4. Enjoy!

### 17. Spinach Spread

Servings: 4
Cooking Time: 10 Minutes
**Ingredients:**
- ½ cup coconut cream
- ¾ cup coconut yogurt
- 10 ounces spinach
- 8 ounces water chestnuts, chopped
- 1 garlic clove, minced

**Directions:**
1. In a pan that fits your Air Fryer, mix coconut cream with spinach, coconut yogurt, chestnuts and garlic, stir, transfer to your Air Fryer, cook at 365 ° F for 10 minutes, blend using an immersion blender, divide into bowls and serve as an appetizer.

### 18. Banana Chips With Black Pepper

Servings: 4
Cooking Time: 10 Minutes
**Ingredients:**
- 4 bananas, peeled and sliced in thin pieces
- A drizzle of olive oil
- A pinch of black pepper

**Directions:**
1. Put banana slices in your air fryer, drizzle the oil, season with pepper, toss to coat gently and cook at 360 degrees for 10 minutes.
2. Serve as a snack.
3. Enjoy!

### 19. Avocado Chips

Servings: 3
Cooking Time: 10 Minutes
**Ingredients:**
- 1 avocado, pitted, peeled and sliced
- Salt and black pepper to the taste
- ½ cup vegan breadcrumbs
- A drizzle of olive oil

**Directions:**

1. In a bowl, mix breadcrumbs with salt and pepper and stir.
2. Brush avocado slices with the oil, coat them in breadcrumbs, place them in your air fryer's basket and cook at 390 degrees F for 10 minutes, shaking halfway.
3. Divide into bowls and serve them as a snack
4. Enjoy!

### 20. Spinach Artichoke Spread

Servings: 8
Cooking Time: 20 Minutes
**Ingredients:**
- 28 ounces canned artichokes, drained and chopped
- 10 ounces spinach
- 8 ounces coconut cream
- 1 yellow onion, chopped
- 2 garlic cloves, minced
- ¾ cup coconut milk
- ½ cup tofu, pressed and crumbled
- 1/3 cup vegan avocado mayonnaise
- 1 tablespoon red vinegar
- A pinch of salt and black pepper

**Directions:**
1. In a pan that fits your air fryer, mix artichokes with spinach, coconut cream, onion, garlic, coconut milk, tofu, avocado mayo, vinegar, salt and pepper, stir well, introduce in the fryer and cook at 365 degrees F for 20 minutes.
2. Divide into bowls and serve as an appetizer.
3. Enjoy!

### 21. Black Bean Burgers

Servings: 4
Cooking Time: 8 Minutes
**Ingredients:**
- Pepper and salt
- 2 cans of black beans (drain one and leave the other undrained)
- 1/2 tomato (Roma variety; diced)
- 1/2 an onion (finely chopped)
- 1/2 cup of panko or breadcrumbs
- 1 teaspoon of cumin (ground)

**Directions:**
1. Get a large bowl and put in the drained black beans. Proceed to mash the beans with a fork. Afterward, empty the undrained can into the bowl and mix together to combine thoroughly.
2. Proceed to introduce the tomatoes, bread or panko crumbs, cumin, and onion into the bowl. Sprinkle with pepper and salt and stir well to mix.
3. Spray the air fryer basket with oil to avoid sticking. Mold the beans mix into patties and put into the air fryer basket. The basket should be able to contain up to 4 parties.
4. Set the temperature and timer of the air fryer to 370 degrees Fahrenheit and eight to ten minutes respectively. Halfway through the cooking time, flip the patties to cook evenly.
5. Serve on plates and enjoy.

### 22. Italian Veggie Appetizer Salad

Servings: 4
Cooking Time: 15 Minutes
**Ingredients:**
- 2 red bell peppers, cut into medium wedges
- 1 sweet potato, cut into medium wedges
- 3 zucchinis, sliced
- ½ cup garlic, minced
- 2 tablespoons olive oil
- Salt and black pepper to the taste
- 1 teaspoon Italian seasoning

**Directions:**
1. In your air fryer's pan, mix bell peppers with sweet potato, zucchinis, garlic, oil, salt, pepper and seasoning, toss, transfer to your air fryer and cook at 365 degrees F for 15 minutes
2. Divide into small bowls and serve cold as an appetizer.
3. Enjoy!

### 23. Cheesy Jalapeno Poppers

Servings: 4
Cooking Time: 5 Minutes
**Ingredients:**
- 6 oz vegan cheddar cheese
- 6 oz dairy free cream cheese
- 8 jalapeno peppers, halved lengthwise and seeded
- Freshly ground black pepper to taste

**Directions:**
1. Mix the vegan cheddar cheese and cream cheese in a bowl and fill the

peppers with the mixture. Sprinkle with some black pepper.
2. Preheat the air fryer and place the peppers in the fryer basket without overlapping.
3. Bake at 350 F for 5 minutes.
4. When ready, serve with sweet dipping sauce.

### 24. Cinnamon Carrot Dip

Servings: 6
Cooking Time: 15 Minutes
**Ingredients:**
- 4 tablespoons olive oil
- 2 cups carrot, grated
- ½ teaspoon cinnamon powder
- Salt and black pepper to the taste
- A pinch of cayenne pepper
- 1 tablespoon chives, chopped

**Directions:**
1. In a pan that fits the fryer, combine oil with carrots, cinnamon, salt, pepper and cayenne, stir, introduce in the fryer and cook at 365 degrees F for 15 minutes.
2. Add chives, stir really well, divide into bowls and serve cold as a dip
3. Enjoy!

### 25. Ancho Chili Dip

Servings: 8
Cooking Time: 12 Minutes
**Ingredients:**
- 5 ancho chilies, dried, seedless and chopped
- 2 garlic cloves, crushed
- Salt and black pepper to the taste
- ½ cups water
- 1 and ½ teaspoons stevia
- ½ teaspoon oregano, dried
- ½ teaspoon cumin, ground
- 2 tablespoons apple cider vinegar

**Directions:**
1. In a pan that fits your air fryer pot mix water with chilies, garlic, salt, pepper, stevia, cumin and oregano, stir, introduce in your air fryer and cook at 365 degrees F for 12 minutes.
2. Transfer this mix to your blender, add vinegar, pulse well, divide into bowls and serve cold.
3. Enjoy!

### 26. Cauliflower Crackers

Servings: 12
Cooking Time: 25 Minutes
**Ingredients:**
- 1 big cauliflower head, florets separated and riced
- ½ cup cashew cheese, shredded
- 1 tablespoon flax meal mixed with 1 tablespoon water
- 1 teaspoon Italian seasoning
- Salt and black pepper to the taste

**Directions:**
1. Spread cauliflower rice on a lined baking sheet that fits your air fryer, introduce in the fryer and cook at 360 degrees F for 10 minutes.
2. Transfer cauliflower to a bowl, add salt, pepper, cashew cheese, flax meal and Italian seasoning, stir really well, spread this into a rectangle pan that fits your air fryer, press well, introduce in the fryer and cook at 360 degrees F for 15 minutes more.
3. Cut into medium crackers and serve as a snack.
4. Enjoy!

### 27. Olives And Eggplant Dip

Servings: 6
Cooking Time: 10 Minutes
**Ingredients:**
- 2 pounds eggplant, sliced
- Salt and black pepper to the taste
- 1 tablespoon olive oil
- 4 garlic cloves, chopped
- ½ cup water
- Juice of 1 lemon
- ¼ cup black olives, pitted
- 1 tablespoon sesame paste
- 4 thyme springs, chopped

**Directions:**
1. In a pan that fits your air fryer, combine oil with eggplants, salt, pepper, garlic, water, lemon juice, olives and thyme, stir, introduce in your fryer and cook at 370 degrees F for 10 minutes.
2. Blend your dip with an immersion blender, add sesame paste, blend again, divide into bowls and serve.
3. Enjoy!

## 28. Eggplant And Tomato Salad

Servings: 4
Cooking Time: 20 Minutes
**Ingredients:**
- 1 and ½ cups tomatoes, chopped
- 3 cups eggplant, cubed
- 6 ounces black olives, pitted and sliced
- 2 teaspoons balsamic vinegar
- 1 tablespoon oregano, chopped
- Salt and black pepper to the taste

**Directions:**
1. In a pan that fits your air fryer, mix tomatoes with eggplant, olives, vinegar, oregano, salt and pepper, toss, introduce in your fryer and cook at 370 degrees F for 20 minutes
2. Divide between small appetizer plates and serve as an appetizer.
3. Enjoy!

## 29. Squash Pate

Servings: 4
Cooking Time: 25 Minutes
**Ingredients:**
- 2 cups butternut squash, peeled and cubed
- 3 tablespoons coconut milk
- A pinch of rosemary, dried
- A pinch of sage, dried
- A pinch of salt and black pepper

**Directions:**
1. In your Air Fryer's pan, mix squash, coconut milk, sage, rosemary, salt and pepper, toss, introduce in your Air Fryer and cook at 375 ° F for 25 minutes.
2. Blend using an immersion blender, divide into bowls and serve cold.

## 30. Creamy Spinach Spread

Servings: 4
Cooking Time: 10 Minutes
**Ingredients:**
- ½ cup coconut cream
- ¾ cup coconut yogurt
- 10 ounces spinach
- 8 ounces water chestnuts, chopped
- 1 garlic clove, minced

**Directions:**
1. In a pan that fits your air fryer, mix coconut cream with spinach, coconut yogurt, chestnuts and garlic, stir, transfer to your air fryer, cook at 365 degrees F for 10 minutes, blend using an immersion blender, divide into bowls and serve as an appetizer.
2. Enjoy!

## 31. Tofu Satay

Servings: 4
Cooking Time: 15 minutes
**Ingredients:**
- 2 garlic cloves
- Juice from 1 fresh line
- A batch of 5-Minute Peanut Butter Sauce (Use the complete 6 cups of water as required by the recipe)
- 1 tsp of Sriracha sauce
- 1 tbsp of maple syrup
- 1 block of tofu (slice into strips)
- 2 tbsp of soy sauce
- 2 tsp of fresh ginger (chop coarsely; peeling not necessary)

**Directions:**
1. Get a food processor or blender and proceed to pour in the Sriracha, soy sauce, maple syrup, garlic, and lime juice. Blend into a smooth puree mix.
2. Marinate the tofu for 15 to 30 minutes by pouring the marinade over the cut tofu strips. Soak six bamboo skewers as the tofu marinate. Ensure there's enough water to submerge them.
3. When the time for marinating elapses, get a wire cutter and cut the skewers in halves. This will produce six half-sized skewers. The reason for halving the skewers is that a complete one may not fit into the air fryer basket. Take off any splinters formed by halving the skewers, and proceed to put a tofu strip into each skewer stick. Ensure the uncut side isn't the part you are sticking through the tofu. This will prevent any splinters from going into the tofu.
4. Move the mini-sized tofu skewers into the air fryer basket. Set the timer and temperature to 15 minutes and 370 degrees Fahrenheit respectively. Refrain from shaking the basket while cooking. As the tofu begins to cook, start preparing the 5-Minute Peanut Butter Sauce, if you haven't already made it.

5. When the air fryer timer elapses, the tofu satay is ready to be served.

### 32. Vegan Goat Cheese Bacon Wrapped Dates

Servings:4
Cooking Time:20 Minutes
**Ingredients:**
- 8 Medjool dates, pitted
- 3+ tablespoons Vegan Goat Cheese
- (or your favorite vegan soft cheese)
- Smoky Rich Bacon mixture (recipe follows - first four Ingredients:)
- 2 sheets rice paper

**Directions:**
1. Preheat oven to 350 °F. Line a baking sheet with parchment.
2. Slice date lengthwise (if your dates are already pitted, look for the slice already made). Fill each date with goat cheese (about one teaspoon each).
3. Using kitchen scissor, cut rice paper into strips as wide as a Medjool date. Hold single strip under water faucet running cool water, just until it begins to soften. Dip strip into cashew butter mixture until well coated, wrap around filled date. Repeat with all dates.
4. Make bacon strips with remaining rice paper (I had three strips left).
5. Bake at 350 °F for 15-18 minutes. Serve warm.
6. These can be made ahead and popped into the oven right before a party!

### 33. Plum And Apple Spread

Servings: 20
Cooking Time: 15 Minutes
**Ingredients:**
- 3 pounds plumps, pitted and chopped
- 2 onions, chopped
- 2 apples, cored and chopped
- 4 tablespoons ginger powder
- 4 tablespoons cinnamon powder
- 1-pint vinegar
- ¾ pound coconut sugar

**Directions:**
1. Put plumps, apples and onions in a pan that fits your air fryer, add ginger, cinnamon, sugar and vinegar, stir, introduce in the fryer and cook at 365 degrees F for 16 minutes.

2. Stir really well, divide into bowls and serve cold as a spread.
3. Enjoy!

### 34. Easy Onion And Corn Spread

Servings: 8
Cooking Time: 15 Minutes
**Ingredients:**
- 30 ounces canned corn, drained
- 2 green onions, chopped
- ½ cup coconut cream
- 8 ounces tofu, crumbled
- 1 jalapeno, chopped
- ½ teaspoon chili powder

**Directions:**
1. In a pan that fits your air fryer, mix corn with green onions, coconut cream, tofu, chili powder and jalapeno, stir, transfer to your fryer and cook at 350 degrees F for 15 minutes.
2. Divide into bowls and serve as a dip.
3. Enjoy!

### 35. Green Tomato And Currants Dip

Servings: 12
Cooking Time: 15 Minutes
**Ingredients:**
- 2 pounds green tomatoes, chopped
- 1 white onion, chopped
- ¼ cup currants
- 1 Anaheim chili pepper, chopped
- 4 red chili peppers, chopped
- 2 tablespoons ginger, grated
- ¾ cup coconut sugar

**Directions:**
1. In a pan that fits your air fryer, mix green tomatoes with onion, currants, Anaheim pepper, chili pepper, ginger, sugar and vinegar, stir, introduce in the fryer and cook at 360 degrees F for 15 minutes.
2. Whisk the dip really well, divide it between bowls and serve cold.
3. Enjoy!

### 36. Cinnamon Sweet Sticky Nuts

Servings: 4
Cooking Time: 6 Minutes
**Ingredients:**
- ½ cup raw pecans
- ½ cup raw almonds
- ½ cup raw walnuts

- ½ cup cashew nuts
- 2 tsp cinnamon powder
- 3 tbsp maple syrup
- 1 tsp melted vegan butter

**Directions:**
1. Add all the ingredients to a bowl and mix until properly combined.
2. Pour the nuts in the fryer basket and toast at 350 F for 6 minutes or until the nuts are crunchy. Shake the basket halfway.
3. Transfer the nuts to a bowl; allow cooling for a few minutes, and start crunching.

### 37. Polenta Biscuits

Servings: 4
Cooking Time: 25 Minutes
**Ingredients:**
- 18 ounces cooked polenta roll, cold
- 1 tablespoon olive oil

**Directions:**
1. Cut polenta in medium slices and brush them with the olive oil.
2. Place polenta biscuits into your air fryer and cook at 400 degrees F for 25 minutes, flipping them after 10 minutes.
3. Serve biscuits as a snack.

### 38. Tomato And Apple Dip

Servings: 14
Cooking Time: 21 Minutes
**Ingredients:**
- 2 pounds tomatoes, peeled and chopped
- 1 apple, cored and chopped
- 1 yellow onion, chopped
- 6 ounces sultanas, chopped
- 3 ounces dates, chopped
- 3 teaspoons whole spice
- ½ pint vinegar
- ½ pound coconut sugar

**Directions:**
1. Put tomatoes in a pan that fits your air fryer, add apple, onion, sultanas, dates, whole spice and half of the vinegar, stir, introduce in the fryer and cook at 360 degrees F for 15 minutes.
2. Add the rest of the vinegar and the sugar, stir, cook at 360 degrees F for 6 minutes more, whisk well, divide into bowls and serve cold.
3. Enjoy!

### 39. Potato And Beans Dip

Servings: 10
Cooking Time: 10 Minutes
**Ingredients:**
- 19 ounces canned garbanzo beans, drained
- 1 cup sweet potatoes, peeled and chopped
- ¼ cup sesame paste
- 2 tablespoons lemon juice
- 1 tablespoon olive oil
- 5 garlic cloves, minced
- ½ teaspoon cumin, ground
- 2 tablespoons water
- Salt and white pepper to the taste

**Directions:**
1. Put potatoes in your air fryer's basket, cook them at 360 degrees F for 10 minutes, cool them down, peel, put them in your food processor and pulse well.
2. Add sesame paste, garlic, beans, lemon juice, cumin, water, oil, salt and pepper, pulse again, divide into bowls and serve cold.
3. Enjoy!

### 40. Vegan Air Fryer Buffalo Cauliflower

Servings:4
Cooking Time:25 Minutes
**Ingredients:**
- 1 large head cauliflower
- 1 cup unbleached all-purpose flour
- 1 teaspoon vegan chicken bouillon granules
- ¼ teaspoon cayenne pepper
- ¼ teaspoon chili powder
- ¼ teaspoon paprika
- ¼ teaspoon dried chipotle chile flakes
- 1 cup soy milk
- canola oil spray
- 2 tablespoons nondairy butter
- ½ cup Cayenne Pepper Sauce or your favorite
- 2 cloves garlic, minced

**Directions:**
1. Cut the cauliflower into bite-size pieces. Rinse and drain the cauliflower pieces.
2. Combine the flour, bouillon granules, cayenne, chili powder, paprika, and chipotle flakes in a large bowl. Slowly

whisk in the milk until a thick batter is formed.

3. Spray the air fryer basket with canola oil and preheat the air fryer to 390°F for 10 minutes.
4. While the air fryer is preheating, toss the cauliflower in the batter. Transfer the battered cauliflower to the air fryer basket. Cook for 20 minutes on 390°F. Using tongs, turn the cauliflower pieces at 10 minutes (don't be alarmed if they stick).
5. After turning the cauliflower, heat the butter, hot sauce, and garlic in a small saucepan over medium high heat. Bring the mixture to a boil, reduce the heat to simmer, and cover.
6. Once the cauliflower is cooked, transfer it to a large bowl. Pour the sauce over the cauliflower and toss gently with tongs. Serve immediately.

### 41. Chickpeas Dip

Servings: 10
Cooking Time: 20 Minutes
**Ingredients:**
- 1 cup canned chickpeas, drained and some of the liquid reserved
- 2 tablespoons olive oil
- 1 tablespoon sesame paste
- A pinch of salt and black pepper
- 1 garlic clove, minced
- 1 tablespoon lemon juice
**Directions:**
1. In a pan that fits your Air Fryer mix chickpeas with salt, pepper, lemon juice and oil, stir, transfer to your Air Fryer and cook at 365 ° F for 20 minutes.
2. Transfer chickpeas to a blender, add sesame paste, reserved liquid and garlic, blend well, divide into bowls and serve as a dip

### 42. Tofu Sweet Paprika Snack

Servings: 4
Cooking Time: 20 Minutes
**Ingredients:**
- 12 ounces firm tofu, cubed
- 1 teaspoon sweet paprika
- 1 teaspoon sesame oil
- 1 tablespoon coriander, chopped

- 2 tablespoons coconut aminos
**Directions:**
1. In a bowl, mix paprika with the oil, coriander and aminos, whisk well, add tofu pieces, toss to coat and leave aside for 30 minutes.
2. Transfer tofu cubes to your air fryer's basket and cook at 350 degrees F for 20 minutes shaking halfway.
3. Transfer them to a bowl and serve as a snack.
4. Enjoy!

### 43. Fennel And Cherry Tomatoes Spread

Servings: 6
Cooking Time: 12 Minutes
**Ingredients:**
- 1 fennel bulb, cut into pieces
- 2 pints cherry tomatoes, halved
- ¼ cup veggie stock
- 5 thyme springs, chopped
- 1 tablespoons olive oil
- Salt and black pepper to the taste
**Directions:**
1. In a pan that fits the fryer, combine fennel with tomatoes, stock, thyme, oil, salt and pepper, toss, introduce in the fryer and cook at 365 degrees F for 12 minutes.
2. Mash the mixture a bit using a fork, stir well, divide into bowls and serve cold.
3. Enjoy!

### 44. Simple Fried Ravioli

Servings: 4
Cooking Time: 10 Minutes
**Ingredients:**
- ¼ cup grated vegan parmesan cheese + extra for garnishing
- 2 cups breadcrumbs
- 24 vegan raviolis
- 1 cup vegan buttermilk
**Directions:**
1. In a bowl, combine the vegan parmesan cheese with the breadcrumbs.
2. Preheat the air fryer.
3. Then, dip the raviolis in the buttermilk and coat generously in the breadcrumbs mixture.
4. Place the raviolis into the fryer basket, oil with cooking spray, and fry at 350 F for 10 minutes or until the raviolis are

golden brown and crispy. Shake the basket halfway.
5. When ready, plate the raviolis, sprinkle with some vegan parmesan, and serve with marinara dipping sauce.

## 45. Chickpeas Snack

Servings: 4
Cooking Time: 20 Minutes
**Ingredients:**
- 15 ounces canned chickpeas, drained
- ½ teaspoon cumin, ground
- 1 tablespoon olive oil
- 1 teaspoon smoked paprika
- Salt and black pepper to the taste

**Directions:**
1. In a bowl, mix chickpeas with oil, cumin, paprika, salt and pepper, toss to coat, place them in the fryer's basket, cook at 390 degrees F for 10 minutes and transfer to a bowl.
2. Serve as a snack
3. Enjoy!

## 46. Simple Falafel

Servings: 4
Cooking Time: 13 Minutes
**Ingredients:**
- 2 (15 oz) cans chickpeas, drained and rinsed
- 4 tbsp raw cashews
- 6 garlic cloves
- 1 tbsp cumin powder
- ¾ cup chopped parsley
- 7 tbsp flour
- ½ tsp salt
- 3 tbsp olive oil

**Directions:**
1. Combine all the ingredients into a food processor and blend to have a slightly rough dough.
2. Form 1-inch balls out of the mixture, place on a plate and flatten into discs with your hands.
3. Preheat the air fryer.
4. Arrange a few falafel pieces in the fryer basket and fry at 350 F for 8 minutes. Flip and cook further for 5 minutes.
5. Plate and prepare the remaining falafel dough.
6. Serve with tahini sauce.

## 47. Sweet Potato Nuggets

Servings: 4
Cooking Time: 10 Minutes
**Ingredients:**
- Sweet Potatoes:
- 3 sweet potatoes, boiled and mashed
- ½ tsp chili flakes
- 1 tsp garlic powder
- Salt and freshly ground black pepper to taste
- 3 tbsp grated vegan cheddar cheese
- ½ tsp Italian mixed herbs
- 2 tbsp chopped parsley
- ¼ cup breadcrumbs
- Coating:
- ¼ cup corn flour
- ¼ cup water
- Salt to taste
- ¼ tsp crushed pepper
- 1 cup breadcrumbs

**Directions:**
1. In a bowl, mix the all the sweet potato ingredients and form bite-size oblong balls from the mixture.
2. In another bowl, combine the cornstarch, water, and salt.
3. Mix the crushed pepper with the breadcrumbs in a small bowl and set aside.
4. Preheat the air fryer.
5. Dip some potato balls into the cornstarch mixture and coat in the seasoned breadcrumbs.
6. Place in the fryer basket in a single layer and crisp at 350 F for 8 to 10 minutes or until the nuggets are golden brown.
7. Plate the bites and cook the remaining nuggets.
8. Serve immediately with almond chipotle dip.

## 48. Potato Chips

Servings: 4
Cooking Time: 30 Minutes
**Ingredients:**
- 4 potatoes, scrubbed, peeled and cut into thin strips
- A pinch of sea salt
- 1 tablespoon olive oil
- 2 teaspoons rosemary, chopped

**Directions:**

1. In a bowl, mix potato chips with salt and oil, toss to coat, place them in your air fryer's basket and cook at 330 degrees F for 30 minutes.
2. Divide them into bowls, sprinkle rosemary all over and serve as a snack.
3. Enjoy!

### 49. Cabbage Rolls

Servings: 8
Cooking Time: 25 Minutes
**Ingredients:**
- 2 cups cabbage, chopped
- 2 yellow onions, chopped
- 1 carrot, chopped
- ½ red bell pepper, chopped
- 1-inch piece ginger, grated
- 8 garlic cloves, minced
- Salt and black pepper to the taste
- 1 teaspoon coconut aminos
- 2 tablespoons olive oil
- 10 vegan spring roll sheets
- Cooking spray
- 2 tablespoons corn flour mixed with 1 tablespoon water

**Directions:**
1. Heat up a pan with the oil over medium-high heat, add cabbage, onions, carrots, bell pepper, ginger, garlic, salt, pepper and aminos, stir, cook for 4 minutes and take off heat.
2. Cut each spring roll sheet and cut into 4 pieces.
3. Place 1 tablespoons veggie mix in one corner, roll and fold edges.
4. Repeat this with the rest of the rolls, place them in your air fryer's basket, grease them with cooking oil and cook at 360 degrees F for 10 minutes on each side.
5. Arrange on a platter and serve as an appetizer.
6. Enjoy!

### 50. Veggie Sticks

Servings: 4
Cooking Time: 30 Minutes
**Ingredients:**
- 4 parsnips, cut into thin sticks
- 2 sweet potatoes, cut into sticks
- 4 carrots, cut into sticks
- Salt and black pepper to the taste
- 2 tablespoons rosemary, chopped
- 2 tablespoons olive oil
- A pinch of garlic powder

**Directions:**
1. Put parsnips, sweet potatoes and carrots in a bowl, add oil, garlic powder, salt, pepper and rosemary and toss to coat.
2. Put sweet potatoes in your preheated air fryer, cook them for 10 minutes at 350 degrees F and transfer them to a platter.
3. Add parsnips to your air fryer, cook for 5 minutes and transfer over potato fries.
4. Add carrots, cook for 15 minutes at 350 degrees F, also transfer to the platter.
5. Serve as a snack.
6. Enjoy!

### 51. Bow Tie Pasta Chips

Servings: 2
Cooking Time: 10 minutes
**Ingredients:**
- 1 tablespoon of nutritional yeast
- 1/2 teaspoon of salt
- 1 tablespoon of olive oil (use aquafaba alternatively)
- 2 cups of 152 grams dry whole wheat pasta (for a gluten-free recipe, use brown rice instead)
- 1½ teaspoon of Italian Seasoning Blend

**Directions:**
1. Start by cooking the pasta for half the time as directed by the cooking instructions on the package. Drain the pasta and drizzle with aquafaba or olive oil. Sprinkle salt, Italian seasoning, and nutritional yeast. Toss thoroughly to mix.
2. Depending on the volume capacity of your air fryer model, you can either place all of the pasta in the basket at once or cook in batches.
3. Set the timer for five minutes and set the temperature to 390 degrees Fahrenheit. Once the timer elapses, shake the air fryer basket and run again for three to five minutes until crunchiness is attained.

### 52.  Crispy Tangy Reuben Rolls

Servings:4
Cooking Time:10 Minutes
**Ingredients:**
- 1 (20 ounce) can jackfruit, drained
- ⅓ cup oil free Vegan Thousand Island Dressing, plus more for dipping
- 1 small sweet onion, peeled and diced
- 2 cloves garlic, peeled and minced
- 6-7 thin slices vegan swiss cheese, optional / omit for oil free
- 2 large dill pickles, chopped
- 12-14 vegan wonton wrappers (rice paper wraps for gluten free)

**Directions:**
1. Using forks, shred jackfruit. Combine with Vegan Thousand Island Dressing, set aside to marinate.
2. In a saucepan over medium heat, sauté onion and garlic in a bit of water until softened and translucent. Remove from heat, combine with jackfruit mixture.
3. To assemble rolls: arrange a wrap in a diamond shape, or run a rice paper wrap under water briefly. Place 2 tablespoons jackfruit mixture in bottom corner. Top with one half slice cheese, if using, and one tablespoon chopped pickles. Roll as pictured in this photo.
4. Brush each roll lightly with pickle juice.
5. Oil Free Air Fryer 350 °F. Arrange Crispy Tangy Reuben Rolls in single layer.
6. Cook for 5 minutes. Remove and turn rolls / shake basket. Return to air fryer for another 3 minutes, or until crisp and golden brown.
7. Baking instructions: preheat oven to 350 °F. Arrange rolls in single layer on baking sheet lined with parchment. Bake at 350 °F for 7 minutes. Remove from oven and turn. Return to oven for another 5-7 minutes, or until crisp and golden brown.
8. Alternatively, an oil-frying option: heat 1-2 tablespoons oil in pan over medium heat, add 3-4 rolls at a time, turning frequently so they get an even light brown crunchiness all around. Remove to a drying rack or paper towel.
9. Serve warm with Vegan Thousand Island Dressing.

### 53.  Chinese Bowls With Tofu

Servings: 4
Cooking Time: 15 Minutes
**Ingredients:**
- 12 ounces firm tofu, cubed
- 3 tablespoons maple syrup
- ¼ cup coconut aminos
- 2 tablespoons sesame oil
- 2 tablespoons lime juice
- 1 pound fresh romanesco, roughly chopped
- 3 carrots, chopped
- 1 red bell pepper, chopped
- 8 ounces spinach, torn
- 2 cup red quinoa, cooked

**Directions:**
1. In a bowl, mix tofu cubes with oil, maple syrup, coconut aminos and lime juice, toss, transfer everything to your air fryer and cook at 370 degrees F for 15 minutes, shaking often.
2. Add romanesco, carrots, spinach, bell pepper and quinoa, toss, divide into bowls and serve.
3. Enjoy!

### 54.  Tofu & "sausage" Sandwich

Servings: 2
Cooking Time: 13 Minutes
**Ingredients:**
- 2 vegan bagels, sliced in half
- 2 vegan breakfast sausages
- ½ teaspoon oil
- 4 thin slices tofu
- Salt and pepper to taste
- ¼ teaspoon nutritional yeast flakes, divided
- ¼ teaspoon granulated onion, divided
- 2 tablespoons vegan cream cheese

**Directions:**
1. Toast the bagels in your toaster until golden.
2. Set aside.
3. Air fry the sausages at 400 degrees F for 10 minutes, flipping once halfway through.
4. In a pan over medium heat, add the oil.
5. Sprinkle salt, pepper, nutritional yeast flakes and onion on both sides.

6. Cook the tofu until golden on both sides.
7. Spread cream cheese on the bagel and top with the sausage and tofu.
8. Place the other bagel slice on top.

## 55. Cocoa Chia Pudding

Servings: 4
Cooking Time: 15 Minutes
**Ingredients:**
- 1 cup chia seeds
- 2 cups coconut milk
- 2 tablespoons coconut, shredded and unsweetened
- ¼ cup maple syrup
- ½ teaspoon cinnamon powder
- 2 teaspoons cocoa powder
- ½ teaspoon vanilla extract

**Directions:**
1. In your air fryer, mix chia seeds, coconut milk, coconut, maple syrup, cinnamon, cocoa powder and vanilla, toss, cover and cook at 365 degrees F for 15 minutes
2. Divide Cocoa Chia Pudding into bowls and serve for breakfast.
3. Enjoy!

## 56. Potatoes With Coconut Cream

Servings: 4
Cooking Time: 20 Minutes
**Ingredients:**
- 1 an ½ pounds potatoes, peeled and cubed
- 2 tablespoons olive oil
- Salt and black pepper to the taste
- 1 tablespoon hot paprika
- 3.5 ounces coconut cream

**Directions:**
1. Put potatoes in a bowl, add water to cover, leave them aside for 10 minutes, drain them, mix with half of the oil, salt, pepper and the paprika and toss them.
2. Put potatoes in your air fryer's basket and cook at 360 degrees F for 20 minutes.
3. In a bowl, mix coconut cream with salt, pepper and the rest of the oil and stir well.
4. Divide potatoes between plates, add coconut cream on top and serve for breakfast
5. Enjoy!

## 57. French Fries

Servings: 1
Cooking Time: 30 Minutes
**Ingredients:**
- 250 grams (9 ounces) potato
- 1 teaspoon coconut oil

**Directions:**
1. Wash the potatoes clean. Leave unpeeled or peel them, if preferred, and then cut into fries.
2. Toss the potato pieces with the coconut oil. Set the temperature to 160C or 320F and set the timer for 20-25 minutes. Halfway through cooking, shake the basket, set the temperature to 180C, and continue cooking.

## 58. "bacon" Breakfast

Servings: 2
Cooking Time: 25 Minutes
**Ingredients:**
- 2 tablespoons tamari
- 1 tablespoon sesame oil, toasted
- 1 tablespoon olive oil
- 1 teaspoon maple syrup
- 1 teaspoon lemon juice
- 1 teaspoon paprika
- Salt and pepper to taste
- ¼ teaspoon vegan Worcestershire sauce
- ½ teaspoon cumin
- 1 medium eggplant, cut into long thin slices
- 2 tablespoons vegan mayonnaise
- 2 vegan muffins
- 4 tomato slices
- 4 cucumber slices

**Directions:**
1. Preheat your air fryer to 300 degrees F.
2. In a bowl, mix the tamari, oils, maple syrup, lemon juice, paprika, salt, pepper, Worcestershire sauce and cumin.
3. Brush both sides of eggplant slice with the mixture.
4. Arrange the eggplant slices on a single layer on the air fryer pan.
5. Cook for 15 minutes or until brown.
6. Spread mayo on the muffin and put the "bacon" on top.
7. Top with the cucumber and tomato slices.

## 59. Vegan Breakfast Sandwich

Servings: 4
Cooking Time: 10 Minutes
**Ingredients:**
- For making the Tofu egg:
- A dash of paprika
- 1/4 cup of soy sauce (light variety)
- 1/2 tsp of turmeric
- 1 block of tofu (extra firm variety. Press and slice into 4 cutlets. Proceed to cut into circles. You can use a biscuit cutter.)
- 1 tsp of garlic powder
- For making the sandwich:
- Any vegan cheese of your choice (cut into 4 slices)
- 4 vegan muffins (English variety): Be careful when shopping for these as popular brands tend to make use of non-vegan milk in making English muffins. Brands found in food stores are likely to stock vegan varieties.
- Tomato and onions (cut into slices.): Optional additions
- 1 Haas avocado (peel and slice)
- Vegan mayonnaise (vegan butter can also be used for this recipe.): Optional addition.

**Directions:**
1. Start by letting the tofu marinate overnight.
2. Get a shallow dish and pour in the soy sauce. Add the tofu, as well as the paprika, turmeric, and garlic powder, and toss together to mix thoroughly.
3. To cook the tofu, set the air fryer to 10 minutes at a temperature of 400 degrees Fahrenheit. Put in the marinated tofu mix into the air fryer and cook. Pause to shake the mix every five minutes.
4. To make the sandwich, spread the vegan butter or vegan mayonnaise on the English muffins. Place the vegan cheese and avocado on top of each other alongside any other toppings of your choosing.
5. When the tofu is well cooked, proceed to include it in the sandwich. Close up the muffin and serve.

## 60. Gorgeous Granola

Servings:4
Cooking Time: 40 Minutes Bake: 248°f
**Ingredients:**
- 1 cup rolled oats
- 3 tablespoons maple syrup
- 1 tablespoon coconut sugar
- 1 tablespoon neutral-flavored oil (such as refined coconut, sunflower, or safflower)
- ¼ teaspoon sea salt
- ¼ teaspoon cinnamon
- ¼ teaspoon vanilla

**Directions:**
1. In a medium-size bowl, stir together the oats, maple syrup, coconut sugar, oil, salt, cinnamon, and vanilla until thoroughly combined. Place in a 6-inch round, 2-inch deep baking pan and bake for 10 minutes.
2. Remove, stir well, and cook for another 10 minutes. Repeat this step, removing and stirring every 10 minutes, for a total of 40 minutes, or until the granola is lightly browned and mostly dry. It won't be totally crisp yet, but will become crisp once it is transferred to a plate and allowed to cool.
3. Store in an airtight container once it's completely cooled and crisp. The granola should keep for at least a week or two in a cool, dry place.

## 61. Mixed Seed Bread

Servings: 4
Cooking Time: 15 Minutes
**Ingredients:**
- Flax Egg:
- 3 tbsp ground flax seeds + 9 tbsp water 5 slices mozzarella cheese
- Bread Batter:
- 1 ½ cups all-purpose flour
- 3 tsp baking powder
- ½ cup chia seeds
- 1 tsp hemp seeds
- 5 tbsp sesame seeds
- 1 tsp ground caraway seeds
- 1 tsp salt
- 2/3 cup dairy free cream cheese, room temperature
- ½ cup melted vegan butter

- ¾ cup coconut cream
- Poppy seeds for sprinkling
- Pumpkin seeds for topping

**Directions:**
1. Whisk the flaxseed powder with water, and allow soaking for 5 minutes.
2. In a bowl, mix all the dry ingredients.
3. Then in another bowl, whisk all the wet ingredients as well as the flax egg using an electric hand mixer.
4. Combine both mixtures while still mixing with the electric hand mixer.
5. Line a loaf pan with parchment paper (a container that can fit into the fryer basket) and preheat the air fryer.
6. Pour the dough into the pan, sprinkle with the poppy and pumpkin seeds, and place in the fryer basket.
7. Bake at 370 F for 15 minutes or until a knife inserted into the bread comes out clean.
8. Remove the food with the parchment paper, allow cooling on a wire rack, and slice.
9. Add the bread to your breakfast options and enjoy.

### 62.  Tofu And Broccoli Bowls

Servings: 4
Cooking Time: 15 Minutes
**Ingredients:**
- 1 block firm tofu, pressed and cubed
- 1 teaspoon rice vinegar
- 2 tablespoons coconut aminos
- 1 tablespoon olive oil
- 1 cup quinoa, cooked
- 4 cups broccoli florets
- 2 tablespoons vegan avocado pesto

**Directions:**
1. In a bowl, mix tofu cubes with vinegar, coconut aminos, oil and broccoli, toss and leave aside for 10 minutes.
2. Transfer tofu to your air fryer's basket and cook at 400 degrees F for 10 minutes.
3. Add broccoli, cover fryer again and cook for 5 minutes more.
4. Divide quinoa into bowls, add tofu and broccoli, top with avocado pesto and serve for breakfast.
5. Enjoy!

### 63.  Apple Cobbler Oatmeal

Servings:2
Cooking Time: 20 Minutes Bake: 392°f
**Ingredients:**
- De-Light-Full Caramelized Apples
- ¾ cup rolled oats (see Ingredient Tip)
- 1½ cups water
- Nondairy vanilla-flavored milk of your choice, unsweetened
- ½ cup granola, or Gorgeous Granola

**Directions:**
1. Make the De-Light-Full Caramelized Apples recipe.
2. Once the apples have been cooking for about ten minutes, begin making the oatmeal: In a medium pot, bring the oats and water to a boil, and then reduce to low heat. Simmer, stirring often, until all of the water is absorbed.
3. Place the oatmeal into two bowls. Pour a small amount of nondairy milk on top.
4. Once done, add the cooked apples on top of the oatmeal, and top with granola. Eat while warm.

### 64.  Greek Veggie With Thyme

Servings: 4
Cooking Time: 45 Minutes
**Ingredients:**
- 8 ounces eggplant, sliced
- 8 ounces zucchini, sliced
- 8 ounces bell peppers, chopped
- 2 garlic cloves, minced
- 5 tablespoons olive oil
- 1 bay leaf
- 1 thyme spring
- 2 onions, chopped
- 8 ounces tomatoes, cut into quarters
- Salt and black pepper to the taste

**Directions:**
1. Heat up a pan that fits your air fryer with 2 tablespoons oil over medium-high heat, add eggplant, salt and pepper, stir, cook for 5 minutes and transfer to a bowl.
2. Heat up the pan with 1 more tablespoon oil, add zucchini, cook for 3 minutes and transfer over eggplant pieces.
3. Heat up the pan again, add bell peppers, stir, cook for 2 minutes and pour over the other veggies.

4. Heat up the pan with 2 tablespoons oil, add onions, stir and cook for 3 minutes.
5. Add tomatoes, the rest of the veggies, bay leaf, thyme, garlic, salt and pepper, stir, transfer to your air fryer and cook at 300 degrees F for 30 minutes.
6. Divide between plates and serve for breakfast.
7. Enjoy!

### 65. Banana And Walnuts Oats

Servings: 4
Cooking Time: 15 Minutes
**Ingredients:**
- 1 banana, peeled and mashed
- 1 cup steel cut oats
- 2 cups almond milk
- 2 cups water
- ¼ cup walnuts, chopped
- 2 tablespoons flaxseed meal
- 2 teaspoons cinnamon powder
- 1 teaspoon vanilla extract
- ½ teaspoon nutmeg, ground

**Directions:**
1. In your air fryer mix oats with almond milk, water, walnuts, flaxseed meal, cinnamon, vanilla and nutmeg, stir, cover and cook at 360 degrees F for 15 minutes.
2. Divide into bowls and serve for breakfast.
3. Enjoy!

### 66. Mung Bean "quiche" With Lime Garlic Sauce

Servings:2
Cooking Time: 15 Minutes Bake: 392°f
**Ingredients:**
- For the lime garlic sauce
- 2 teaspoons tamari or shoyu
- 1 teaspoon fresh lime juice
- 1 large garlic clove, minced or pressed
- Dash red chili flakes
- For the "quiche"
- ½ cup mung beans
- ½ cup water
- ¼ teaspoon sea salt
- ⅛ teaspoon freshly ground black pepper
- ½ cup minced onion
- 1 scallion, trimmed and chopped

- Cooking oil spray (sunflower, safflower, or refined coconut)

**Directions:**
1. Soak the mung beans in plenty of water to cover overnight, or for about 8 hours. Drain the mung beans, rinse, and set aside.
2. Preheat the air fryer with the 6-inch round, 2-inch deep baking pan inside for 2 minutes.
3. Place the soaked, drained beans in a blender with the water, salt, and pepper. Blend until smooth. Stir in the onion and scallion, but do not blend.
4. Spray the preheated pan with a little oil spray and pour the batter into the oiled pan. Bake for 15 minutes, or until golden-browned and a knife inserted in the center comes out clean.
5. Once cooked through, cut the "quiche" into quarters and serve drizzled with the sauce.

### 67. Tomatoes Breakfast Salad

Servings: 2
Cooking Time: 20 Minutes
**Ingredients:**
- 2 tomatoes, halved
- Cooking spray
- Salt and black pepper to the taste
- 1 teaspoon parsley, chopped
- 1 teaspoon basil, chopped
- 1 teaspoon oregano, chopped
- 1 teaspoon rosemary, chopped
- 1 cucumber, chopped
- 1 green onion, chopped

**Directions:**
1. Spray tomato halves with cooking oil, season with salt and pepper, place them in your air fryer's basket and cook at 320 degrees F for 20 minutes.
2. Transfer tomatoes to a bowl, add parsley, basil, oregano, rosemary, cucumber and onion, toss and serve for breakfast.
3. Enjoy!

### 68. Roasted Tofu Broccoli Bowl With Quinoa

Servings: 4
Cooking Time: 15-17 Minutes
**Ingredients:**
- For the broccoli-tofu bowl:

- 1 1/4 cups water, plus more if needed for cooking the quinoa
- 1 block tofu, extra firm, pressed and then sliced into 1-inch cubes
- 1 cup quinoa
- 1 tablespoon olive oil
- 1 teaspoon rice vinegar
- 2 tablespoons soy sauce
- 4 cups broccoli florets
- 4 cups water
- Oil-free vegan avocado pesto, ingredient and directions follow
- For the oil-free vegan avocado pesto:
- 1 cup raw cashews
- 2 fresh lemons, juice only
- 2 Haas avocados, peels and pits removed, avocado meat chopped into pieces
- 2 packed cups fresh basil leaves
- 4 cloves garlic
- Salt and pepper, to taste

**Directions:**
1. For the broccoli-tofu bowl:
2. Put the tofu into a large-sized, shallow dish. Add the vinegar, soy sauce, and 1 tablespoon olive oil and toss to coat. Set aside and let marinate for at least 20 minutes.
3. While the tofu is marinating, cook the quinoa with the 1 1/4 cups of water using the method of your choice.
4. Meanwhile, pour 4 cups water into a small-sized pan and bring to a boil over high heat. When the water is boiling, drop the broccoli in the water and cook for 2 minutes – don't bring back to a boil; start counting down as soon as you drop the broccoli in the hot water. After 2 minutes, immediately strain the broccoli in a colander set in the sink. Rinse immediately with cold water to stop cooking.
5. Transfer the marinated tofu into the air fryer basket- reserve any marinade left in the bowl. Set the temperature to 400F and the timer for 10 minutes – shake after 7 minutes.
6. Meanwhile, add the reserved marinade into the bowl with broccoli and toss to coat.
7. After the 10 minutes of tofu cooking time is over, add the broccoli to the air

fryer and cook at 400F for 5 to 7 minutes.
8. Divide the quinoa between 4 serving bowls and divide the broccoli-tofu mixture between the bowls. Drizzle the top with the pesto or your preferred sauce.
9. For the oil-free vegan avocado pesto:
10. Put all of the ingredients in a blender and blend until smooth – add 1 tablespoon water at a time as needed to get the ingredients moving. Season with pepper and salt to taste.
11. You can use this as a sandwich spread, over pasta, or with veggies or bread.
12. Notes: You can make the pesto while the broccoli and tofu cook. Use any sauce if you do not like pesto.

### 69. Vanilla And Cinnamon Porridge

Servings: 4
Cooking Time: 16 Minutes
**Ingredients:**
- 3 cups brown rice, cooked
- 1 and ¾ cups almond milk
- 2 tablespoons coconut sugar
- 2 tablespoons flaxseed meal
- 2 tablespoons raisins
- ¼ teaspoon cinnamon powder
- ¼ teaspoon vanilla extract

**Directions:**
1. In your air fryer, mix rice, milk, sugar, flax meal, raisins, cinnamon and vanilla, stir, cover and cook at 360 degrees F for 16 minutes.
2. Stir porridge again, divide into bowls and serve for breakfast.
3. Enjoy!

### 70. Breakfast Frittata

Servings: 2
Cooking Time: 20 Minutes
**Ingredients:**
- Cooking spray
- ¼ lb. breakfast sausage, cooked and crumbled
- 4 vegan eggs
- ½ cup vegan cheese
- 2 tablespoons red bell pepper, diced
- 1 green onion, chopped

**Directions:**
1. Spray oil on a small cake pan.

2. Preheat your air fryer to 360 degrees F.
3. Combine all the ingredients in a bowl.
4. Pour the mixture into the cake pan.
5. Cook in the air fryer for 20 minutes.

### 71. Breakfast Sandwich

Servings: 4
Cooking Time: 10 Minutes
**Ingredients:**
- ½ teaspoon turmeric
- 1 teaspoon garlic powder
- ¼ cup light soy sauce
- Paprika to taste
- 4 slices tofu, cut into rounds using cookie cutter
- 4 vegan English muffins, sliced in half
- 4 teaspoons vegan mayonnaise
- 1 avocado, sliced
- 4 slices vegan cheese
- 4 white onion rings
- 4 slices tomato

**Directions:**
1. In a bowl, mix turmeric, garlic powder, soy sauce and paprika.
2. Marinate tofu rounds for 10 minutes.
3. Cook in the air fryer at 400 degrees F for 10 minutes, shaking once halfway through.
4. Spread the mayo on the muffin and put the avocado and cheese on top.
5. Put the tofu above the cheese.
6. Top with onion ring and tomato slice.
7. Place the other half of the muffin on top.

### 72. Veggie Casserole With Tofu

Servings: 2
Cooking Time: 15 Minutes
**Ingredients:**
- 1 yellow onion, chopped
- 1 teaspoon garlic, minced
- 1 teaspoon olive oil
- 1 carrot, chopped
- 2 celery stalks, chopped
- ½ cup shiitake mushrooms, chopped
- ½ cup red bell pepper, chopped
- Salt and black pepper to the taste
- 1 teaspoon oregano, dried
- ½ teaspoon red pepper flakes
- ½ teaspoon cumin, ground
- ½ teaspoon dill, dried
- 7 ounces firm tofu, cubed

- 1 tablespoon lemon juice
- 2 tablespoons water
- ½ cup quinoa, already cooked
- 2 tablespoons nutritional yeast

**Directions:**
1. Heat up a pan with the oil over medium-high heat, add garlic and onion, stir and cook for 3 minutes.
2. Add bell pepper, celery and carrot, stir and cook for 3 minutes.
3. Add salt, pepper, mushrooms, oregano, dill, cumin and pepper flakes, stir and cook for 3 minutes more.
4. In your food processor, mix tofu with yeast, lemon juice and water and blend well.
5. Add quinoa and blend again.
6. Add sautéed veggies, stir gently pour everything into your air fryer's pan and cook everything at 350 degrees F for 15 minutes.
7. Divide your breakfast casserole between plates and serve.
8. Enjoy!

### 73. Almond And Cranberry Quinoa

Servings: 4
Cooking Time: 13 Minutes
**Ingredients:**
- 1 cup quinoa
- 3 cups coconut water
- 1 teaspoon vanilla extract
- 3 teaspoons stevia
- 1/8 cup coconut flakes
- ¼ cup cranberries, dried
- 1/8 cup almonds, chopped

**Directions:**
1. In your air fryer, mix quinoa with coconut water, vanilla, stevia, coconut flakes, almonds and cranberries, toss, cover and cook at 365 degrees F for 13 minutes.
2. Divide into bowls and serve for breakfast.
3. Enjoy!

### 74. Air-grilled Tomatoes

Servings: 2
Cooking Time: 20 Minutes
**Ingredients:**
- 2 tomatoes
- Your preferred herbs

- Ground black pepper, such as sage, rosemary, thyme, basil, oregano, parsley, etc.
- Cooking spray

**Directions:**
1. Wash the tomatoes clean and then slice into halves. Spray both sides of the tomatoes with1 spray cooking spray. Sprinkle the cut portion with black pepper and your choice of fresh or dried herbs.
2. With the cut side faced up, put the tomato halves in the air fryer basket. Set the temperature to 160C and the timer for 20 minutes.
3. When the timer beeps, check the doneness, and if needed, cook for a couple of minutes. Cooking time will vary on the size and ripeness of the tomatoes and your preference.
4. Serve them piping hot, at room temperature, or chilled as part of an antipasto.

### 75. Black Bean Totchos With Garlic Lemon Sauce

Servings:4
Cooking Time:15 Minutes
**Ingredients:**
- 1¼ cups tater tots
- 1 cup black beans
- salsa
- sour cream (dairy free / vegan)
- garlic lemon sauce

**Directions:**
1. Prepare air fryer if using. Set temp to 400 °F, cook tater tots for 7 minutes. Remove, shake to turn tater tots, add edamame. Return to air fryer and cook another 5 minutes, until tots are completely cooked through and edamame is hot.
2. Preheat oven to 425 °F if using oven. Line baking sheet with parchment.
3. On a prepared (parchment) baking sheet, arrange tater tots in a single layer. Bake for 15 minutes, remove reduce oven temperature to 375 °F. Using a spatula, flip tater tots and keeping in single layer, move to one side of baking sheet.
4. While tater tots bake, prepare garlic lemon sauce, slice green onion and prep toppings.
5. Assemble totchos: on two plates, pile tots, black beans, salsa, sour cream and garlic lemon sauce. Top with green onion, serve immediately.

### 76. Onion Appetizers

Servings: 4
Cooking Time: 4 Minutes
**Ingredients:**
- 2 lb. onions, sliced into rings
- 2 vegan eggs
- 1 cup almond milk
- 2 cups flour
- 1 tablespoon paprika
- Salt and pepper to taste
- 1 teaspoon garlic powder
- 1 teaspoon cayenne pepper
- Cooking spray
- ¼ cup vegan mayo
- ¼ cup vegan sour cream
- 1 tablespoon ketchup

**Directions:**
1. Combine the eggs and milk in one plate.
2. In another plate, mix the flour, paprika, salt, pepper, garlic powder and cayenne pepper.
3. Dip each onion into the egg mixture before coating with the flour mixture.
4. Spray with oil.
5. Air fryer at 350 degrees F for 4 minutes or until golden and crispy.
6. Serve with the dipping sauces.

### 77. Breakfast Tofu Scramble

Servings: 3
Cooking Time: 30 Minutes
**Ingredients:**
- 1 teaspoon turmeric
- 2 tablespoons soy sauce
- ½ teaspoon onion powder
- ½ teaspoon garlic powder
- ½ cup onion, chopped
- 2 tablespoons olive oil, divided
- 1 block tofu, cubed
- 2 ½ cups potato, cubed

**Directions:**
1. In a bowl, combine the turmeric, soy sauce, onion powder, garlic powder, onion and half of the olive oil.

2. Marinate the tofu cubes in the mixture for 10 minutes.
3. In another bowl, coat the potato cubes with the remaining olive oil.
4. Cook the potatoes in the air fryer at 400 degrees F for 15 minutes, shaking halfway through.
5. Add the tofu and cook at 370 degrees F for another 15 minutes.

### 78. Avocado Rolls

Servings: 5
Cooking Time: 25 Minutes
**Ingredients:**
- 10 rice paper wrappers
- 3 avocados, sliced
- 1 tomato, diced
- Salt and pepper to taste
- 1 tablespoon olive oil
- 4 tablespoons sriracha
- 2 tablespoons sugar
- 1 tablespoon rice vinegar
- 1 tablespoon sesame oil

**Directions:**
1. Mash avocados in a bowl.
2. Stir in the tomatoes, salt and pepper.
3. Mix well.
4. Arrange the rice paper wrappers.
5. Scoop mixture on top.
6. Roll and seal the edges with water.
7. Cook in the air fryer at 350 degrees F for 5 minutes.
8. Mix the rest of the ingredients.
9. Serve rolls with the sriracha dipping sauce.

### 79. Simple Creamy Breakfast Potatoes

Servings: 8
Cooking Time: 20 Minutes
**Ingredients:**
- Cooking spray
- 2 pounds gold potatoes, halved and sliced
- 1 yellow onion, cut into medium wedges
- 10 ounces canned vegan potato cream soup
- 8 ounces coconut milk
- 1 cup tofu, crumbled
- ½ cup veggie stock
- Salt and black pepper to the taste

**Directions:**

1. Grease your air fryer's pan with cooking spray and arrange half of the potatoes on the bottom.
2. Layer onion wedges, half of the vegan cream soup, coconut milk, tofu, stock, salt and pepper.
3. Add the rest of the potatoes, onion wedges, cream, coconut milk, tofu and stock, cover and cook at 365 degrees F for 20 minutes.
4. Divide between plates and serve.
5. Enjoy!

### 80. Delish Donut Holes

Servings:3
Cooking Time: 16 Minutes Fry: 347°f
**Ingredients:**
- 1 tablespoon ground flaxseed
- 1½ tablespoons water
- ¼ cup nondairy milk, unsweetened
- 2 tablespoons neutral-flavored oil (sunflower, safflower, or refined coconut)
- 1½ teaspoons vanilla
- 1½ cups whole-wheat pastry flour or all-purpose gluten-free flour
- ¾ cup coconut sugar, divided
- 2½ teaspoons cinnamon, divided
- ½ teaspoon nutmeg
- ¼ teaspoon sea salt
- ¾ teaspoon baking powder
- Cooking oil spray (refined coconut, sunflower, or safflower)

**Directions:**
1. In a medium bowl, stir the flaxseed with the water and set aside for 5 minutes, or until gooey and thick.
2. Add the milk, oil, and vanilla. Stir well and set this wet mixture aside.
3. In a small bowl, combine the flour, ½ cup coconut sugar, ½ teaspoon cinnamon, nutmeg, salt, and baking powder. Stir very well. Add this mixture to the wet mixture and stir together—it will be stiff, so you'll need to knead it lightly, just until all of the ingredients are thoroughly combined.
4. Spray the air fryer basket with oil. Pull off bits of the dough and roll into balls (about 1 inch in size each). Place in the basket, leaving room in between as they'll increase in size a smidge. (You'll

need to work in batches, as you probably won't be able to cook all 12 at once.) Spray the tops with oil and fry for 6 minutes.

5. Remove the pan, spray the donut holes with oil again, flip them over, and spray them with oil again. Fry them for 2 more minutes, or until golden-brown.
6. During these last 2 minutes of frying, place the remaining 4 tablespoons coconut sugar and 2 teaspoons cinnamon in a bowl, and stir to combine.
7. When the donut holes are done frying, remove them one at a time and coat them as follows: Spray with oil again and toss with the cinnamon-sugar mixture. Spray one last time, and coat with the cinnamon-sugar one last time. Enjoy fresh and warm if possible, as they're best that way.

### 81. French Toast

Servings: 8
Cooking Time: 6 Minutes
**Ingredients:**
- 1 cup pecans
- 2 tablespoons flaxseeds
- 1 teaspoon ground cinnamon
- 1 cup rolled oats
- ¾ cup almond milk
- 8 pieces whole grain vegan bread
- Maple syrup

**Directions:**
1. Pulse pecans, flaxseeds, cinnamon and oats in the food processor until crumbly.
2. Transfer to a dish.
3. In another place, pour in the almond milk.
4. Soak each bread slice for 10 seconds in the almond milk.
5. Dredge with the pecan mixture.
6. Cook the bread in the air fryer at 350 degrees for 3 minutes.
7. Flip the bread and cook for an additional 3 minutes.
8. Drizzle maple syrup on top.

### 82. Kale And Potato Nuggets

Servings:4
Cooking Time:15 Minutes
**Ingredients:**

- 2 cups finely chopped potatoes
- 1 teaspoon extra-virgin olive oil or canola oil
- 1 clove garlic, minced
- 4 cups loosely packed coarsely chopped kale
- ⅛ cup almond milk
- ¼ teaspoon sea salt
- ⅛ teaspoon ground black pepper
- Vegetable oil spray, as needed

**Directions:**
1. Add the potatoes to a large saucepan of boiling water. Cook until tender, about 30 minutes.
2. In a large skillet, heat the oil over medium-high heat. Add the garlic and sauté until golden brown. Add the kale and sauté for 2 to 3 minutes. Transfer to a large bowl.
3. Drain the cooked potatoes and transfer them to a medium bowl. Add the milk, salt, and pepper and mash with a fork or potato masher. Transfer the potatoes to the large bowl and combine with the cooked kale. Preheat the air fryer to 390°F for 5 minutes.
4. Roll the potato and kale mixture into 1-inch nuggets. Spritz the air fryer basket with vegetable oil. Place the nuggets in the air fryer and cook for 12 to 15 minutes, until golden brown, shaking at 6 minutes.

### 83. Crispy Southern Fried Tofu

Servings:4
Cooking Time:25 Minutes
**Ingredients:**
- 1 (14 ounce) block extra firm tofu, drained
- 1 cup vegetable broth
- 1 tablespoon gluten free tamari
- 1¼ cups corn flakes
- 1 tablespoon nutritional yeast
- 1 teaspoon onion powder
- ½ teaspoon celery salt
- ¼ teaspoon smoked paprika
- ¼ teaspoon kala namak, or ½ teaspoon sea salt

**Directions:**
1. Remove tofu from package, drain water. Allow tofu to sit in container several minutes, to continue draining.

2. Do not press tofu. After resting several minutes, pat tofu dry with a paper towel or towel.
3. Slice tofu into slabs or cubes.
4. In shallow bowl / container, combine broth and tamari. Add tofu to broth, arranging in single layer to evenly marinate. Cover and place in refrigerator, several hours to overnight.
5. Preheat oven to 350 °F if using oven. Line a baking sheet with parchment.
6. If using air fryer, prep as normal. I lined the basket with this liner to prevent sticking.
7. Using a blender, food processor, or baggie with a mallet, crush corn flakes to a fine powdery crumb.
8. In a shallow dish, whisk together corn flake crumb, nutritional yeast, onion powder, celery salt, smoked paprika and salt.
9. Take a slab of tofu directly from the marinade and press into crumb, coating each side. Place on lined baking sheet or lined fryer basket. Repeat with each tofu slab.
10. In oven, bake at 350 °F for 10 minutes. Remove from oven, flip tofu to other side, return to oven and bake another 8-10 minutes, until golden and crispy.
11. In air fryer, set to 350 °F and fry for 7 minutes. Remove, flip tofu to other side, return to fryer for another 7 minutes at 350 °F.

### 84. Black Bean Burger

Servings: 6
Cooking Time: 25 Minutes
**Ingredients:**
- 1 ¼ cup rolled oats
- 16 oz. black beans, rinsed and drained
- ¾ cup salsa
- 1 tablespoon soy sauce
- 1 ¼ teaspoons chili powder
- ¼ teaspoon chipotle chili powder
- ½ teaspoon garlic powder

**Directions:**
1. Pulse the oats inside a food processor until powdery.
2. Add all the other ingredients and pulse until well blended.
3. Transfer to a bowl and refrigerate for 15 minutes.

4. Form into burger patties.
5. Cook in the air fryer at 375 degrees F for 15 minutes.

### 85. Potato Hash

Servings: 4
Cooking Time: 40 Minutes
**Ingredients:**
- 750 grams potatoes, washed, peeled or unpeeled, cut into small-sized cubes
- 250 milliliters egg substitute
- 3-5 tablespoons coconut oil, OR vegan fat of choice
- 1/2 teaspoon thyme
- 1/2 teaspoon savory seasoning mixture
- 1/2 teaspoon black pepper
- 1/2 green pepper, washed, seeded, and chopped
- 1 teaspoon salt substitute
- 1 onion, medium-sized, peeled and diced

**Directions:**
1. Preheat the air fryer to 180C.
2. Toss the green pepper and onion with half of the coconut oil and put into the air fryer basket. Set the timer for 5 minutes.
3. Toss the potatoes with the remaining coconut oil and the seasonings. When the air fryer timer beeps, add the potatoes in the air fryer basket, toss the ingredients to mix and cook for 30 minutes. Shake the basket after 15 minutes.
4. While the potato mixture is cooking in the air fryer, lightly grease a nonstick pan with cooking spray. Grind some whole peppers into the pan and let heat for 1 minutes to develop the flavor. Add the egg substitute and cook until solid. Remove from the pan, chop, and set aside.
5. When the air fryer timer beeps, add the egg to the air fryer basket and set the timer for 5 minutes.
6. Serve while piping hot with fresh tomato slices and whatever you want for breakfast.

### 86. Pumpkin Oatmeal

Servings: 4
Cooking Time: 20 Minutes
**Ingredients:**

- 1 and ½ cups water
- ½ cup pumpkin puree
- 1 teaspoon pumpkin pie spice
- 3 tablespoons stevia
- ½ cup steel cut oats

**Directions:**
1. In your air fryer's pan, mix water with oats, pumpkin puree, pumpkin spice and stevia, stir, cover and cook at 360 degrees F for 20 minutes
2. Divide into bowls and serve for breakfast.
3. Enjoy!

### 87. Vegan Cauliflower Chickpea Tacos

Servings: 4.
Cooking Time: 20 minutes.
**Ingredients:**
- 2 tbsp of olive oil
- 4 cups of cauliflower florets. (cut up into bite-sized bits)
- 2 tbsp of taco seasoning
- 19 ounces of chickpeas (rinse and drain)
- For the servings:
- Coconut yogurt (for the drizzle)
- 8 tortillas (small variety)
- 4 cups of cabbage (rinse and shred)
- 2 avocados (washed and sliced)

**Directions:**
1. Place the chopped cauliflower and washed chickpeas into a bowl and spread with the taco seasoning. Toss evenly. For this recipe, you can use a homemade taco seasoning or get one from a food store.
2. Pour the mixed ingredients into the basket of the air fryer. Close and allow to cook for 20 minutes.
3. While cooking, shake the basket regularly to ensure the food is well cooked but not burnt. When the cauliflower attains a perfect brown, turn off the air fryer.
4. Serve in dishes with slices of avocado and shredded cabbage. Drizzle some coconut yogurt for an even better taste.

### 88. Vanilla And Cinnamon Toast

Servings: 6
Cooking Time: 5 Minutes
**Ingredients:**

- A drizzle of vegetable oil
- 12 vegan bread slices
- ½ cup coconut sugar
- A pinch of black pepper
- 1 and ½ teaspoons vanilla extract
- 1 and ½ teaspoons cinnamon powder

**Directions:**
1. In a bowl, mix oil with cinnamon, sugar, vanilla and a pinch of pepper and stir well.
2. Spread this over bread slices, put them in your air fryer, cook at 400 degrees F for 5 minutes, divide them between plates and serve for breakfast
3. Enjoy!

### 89. Blueberry Breakfast Cobbler

Servings:4
Cooking Time: 15 Minutes Bake: 347°f
**Ingredients:**
- ⅓ cup whole-wheat pastry flour
- ¾ teaspoon baking powder
- Dash sea salt
- ⅓ cup unsweetened nondairy milk
- 2 tablespoons maple syrup
- ½ teaspoon vanilla
- Cooking oil spray (sunflower, safflower, or refined coconut)
- ½ cup blueberries
- ¼ cup granola, plain, or Gorgeous Granola
- Nondairy yogurt (for topping, optional)

**Directions:**
1. In a medium bowl, whisk together the flour, baking powder, and salt. Add the milk, maple syrup, and vanilla and whisk gently, just until thoroughly combined.
2. Spray a 6-inch round, 2-inch deep baking pan with cooking oil and pour the mixture into the pan, using a rubber spatula so you don't leave any goodness behind. Top evenly with the blueberries and granola.
3. Place the pan in the air fryer and bake for 15 minutes, or until nicely browned and a knife inserted in the middle comes out clean (aside from gooey blueberries, that is). Enjoy plain or topped with a little nondairy vanilla yogurt. Delish!

### 90. Breakfast-style Potatoes

Servings: 2-4
Cooking Time: 25 Minutes
**Ingredients:**
- 2 Russet potatoes, medium- sized, (about 13 ounces or 2 generous cups total), chopped into roughly 1-inch pieces
- 1 onion, small-sized (about 4 ounces or 3/4 cup), chopped into medium-sized pieces
- 1 bell pepper, small-sized, (about 5 ounces or 3/4 cup), chopped into medium-sized pieces
- A couple generous sprays of cooking oil spray
- Pinch salt and pepper

**Directions:**
1. Put the potatoes in the air fryer basket. Spray with cooking oil spray, shake, spray again, and sprinkle with 1 pinch salt.
2. Set the temperature to 400F and set the timer for 10 minutes. Stop halfway during cooking to shake or stir the potatoes and continue during cooking.
3. When the ten minutes are up, add the onions and bell pepper in the air fryer. Spray with cooking oil and shake the basket. Cook at 400F for another 15 minutes. When there are only 5 minutes left in the cooking time, check the potatoes to ensure that they are not browning too much – cooking time will depend on the size of the potatoes. Add a couple more cooking time, if needed. Season with salt to taste and then serve.

### 91. Noochy Tofu

Servings:4
Cooking Time: 14 Minutes Bake: 392°f
**Ingredients:**
- 1 (8-ounce) package firm or extra-firm tofu
- 4 teaspoons tamari or shoyu
- 1 teaspoon onion granules
- ½ teaspoon garlic granules
- ½ teaspoon turmeric powder
- ¼ teaspoon freshly ground black pepper
- 2 tablespoons nutritional yeast
- 1 teaspoon dried rosemary
- 1 teaspoon dried dill
- 2 teaspoons arrowroot (or cornstarch)
- 2 teaspoons neutral-flavored oil (such as sunflower, safflower, or melted refined coconut)
- Cooking oil spray (sunflower, safflower, or refined coconut)

**Directions:**
1. Cut the tofu into slices and press out the excess water (see Tip).
2. Cut the slices into ½-inch cubes and place in a bowl. Sprinkle with the tamari and toss gently to coat. Set aside for a few minutes.
3. Toss the tofu again, then add the onion, garlic, turmeric, and pepper. Gently toss to thoroughly coat.
4. Add the nutritional yeast, rosemary, dill, and arrowroot. Toss gently to coat.
5. Finally, drizzle with the oil and toss one last time. Spray the air fryer basket with the oil. Place the tofu in the air fryer basket and bake for 7 minutes. Remove, shake gently (so that the tofu cooks evenly), and cook for another 7 minutes, or until the tofu is crisp and browned.

### 92. Roasted Vegetable Tacos

Servings:3
Cooking Time: 12 Minutes Roast: 392°f
**Ingredients:**
- Cooking oil spray (sunflower, safflower, or refined coconut)
- 1 small zucchini
- 1 small-medium yellow onion
- ¼ teaspoon garlic granules
- ⅛ teaspoon sea salt
- Freshly ground black pepper
- 1 (15-ounce) can vegan refried beans
- 6 corn tortillas
- Fresh salsa of your choice
- 1 avocado, cut into slices, or fresh guacamole

**Directions:**
1. Spray the air fryer basket with the oil. Cut the zucchini and onion according to the Cooking Tip that follows and place in the air fryer basket. Spray with more oil and sprinkle evenly with the garlic, salt, and pepper to taste. Roast for 6 minutes. Remove, shake or stir

well, and cook for another 6 minutes, or until the veggies are nicely browned and tender.
2. In a small pan, warm the refried beans over low heat. Stir often. Once to temperature, remove from the heat and set aside.
3. To prepare the tortillas, sprinkle them individually with a little water, then place in a hot skillet (in a single layer; you may need to do this in batches), turning over as each side becomes hot.
4. To make the breakfast tacos: Place a corn tortilla on your plate and fill it with beans, roasted vegetables, salsa, and avocado slices.

### 93. Yam Breakfast Mix

Servings: 4
Cooking Time: 8 Minutes
**Ingredients:**
- 16 ounces canned candied yams, drained
- ½ teaspoon cinnamon powder
- ¼ teaspoon allspice, ground
- ½ cup coconut sugar
- 1 tablespoon flax meal mixed with 2 tablespoons water
- 2 tablespoons coconut cream
- ½ cup maple syrup
- Cooking spray

**Directions:**
1. In a bowl, mix yams with cinnamon and all spice, mash with a fork and stir well.
2. Grease your air fryer with cooking spray, preheat it to 400 degrees F and spread yams mix on the bottom.
3. Add sugar, flax meal, coconut cream and maple syrup, stir gently, cover and cook on for 8 minutes.
4. Divide yams mix between plates and serve for breakfast.
5. Enjoy!

### 94. Delicious Porridge

Servings: 4
Cooking Time: 16 Minutes
**Ingredients:**
- 3 cups brown rice, cooked
- 1 and ¾ cups almond milk
- 2 tablespoons coconut sugar
- 2 tablespoons flaxseed meal

- 2 tablespoons raisins
- ¼ teaspoon cinnamon powder
- ¼ teaspoon vanilla extract

**Directions:**
1. In your air fryer, mix rice, milk, sugar, flax meal, raisins, cinnamon and vanilla, stir, cover and cook at 360 degrees F for 16 minutes.
2. Stir porridge again, divide into bowls and serve for breakfast.
3. Enjoy!

### 95. Mediterranean Chickpeas Breakfast

Servings: 2
Cooking Time: 12 Minutes
**Ingredients:**
- Cooking spray
- 3 shallots, chopped
- 2 garlic cloves, minced
- ½ teaspoon sweet paprika
- ½ teaspoon smoked paprika
- ½ teaspoon cinnamon powder
- Salt and black pepper to the taste
- 2 tomatoes, chopped
- 2 cup chickpeas, cooked
- 1 tablespoon parsley, chopped

**Directions:**
1. Spray your air fryer with cooking spray and preheat it to 365 degrees F.
2. Add shallots, garlic, sweet and smoked paprika, cinnamon, salt, pepper, tomatoes, parsley and chickpeas, toss, cover and cook for 12 minutes.
3. Divide into bowls and serve for breakfast.
4. Enjoy!

### 96. Cinnamon And Apple Oatmeal

Servings: 3
Cooking Time: 15 Minutes
**Ingredients:**
- 3 cups water
- 1 cup steel cut oats
- 1 apple, cored and chopped
- 1 tablespoon cinnamon powder

**Directions:**
1. In your air fryer, mix water with oats, cinnamon and apple, stir, cover and cook at 365 degrees F for 15 minutes.
2. Stir again, divide into bowls and serve for breakfast.
3. Enjoy!

## 97. Veggie Burrito With Tofu

Servings: 8
Cooking Time: 15 Minutes
**Ingredients:**
- 16 ounces tofu, crumbled
- 1 green bell pepper, chopped
- ¼ cup scallions, chopped
- 15 ounces canned black beans, drained
- 1 cup vegan salsa
- ½ cup water
- ¼ teaspoon cumin, ground
- ½ teaspoon turmeric powder
- ½ teaspoon smoked paprika
- A pinch of salt and black pepper
- ¼ teaspoon chili powder
- 3 cups spinach leaves, torn
- 8 vegan tortillas for serving

**Directions:**
1. In your air fryer, mix tofu with bell pepper, scallions, black beans, salsa, water, cumin, turmeric, paprika, salt, pepper and chili powder, stir, cover and cook at 370 degrees F for 20 minutes
2. Add spinach, toss well, divide this on your vegan tortillas, roll, wrap them and serve for breakfast.
3. Enjoy!

## 98. Breakfast Potatoes

Servings: 4
Cooking Time: 25 Minutes
**Ingredients:**
- 2 potatoes, chopped
- 2 teaspoons olive oil
- Salt and pepper to taste
- 1 onion, chopped
- 1 bell pepper, chopped

**Directions:**
1. Toss the potatoes in oil and season with salt and pepper.
2. Cook in the air fryer at 400 degrees F for 10 minutes, shaking once halfway through.
3. Add the onion and bell pepper.
4. Toss to mix and cook for 400 degrees for another 10 to 15 minutes.

## 99. Fruit Crumble

Servings: 2
Cooking Time: 15 Minutes
**Ingredients:**
- 1 apple, diced
- ¼ cup frozen strawberries
- ¼ cup frozen blueberries
- 2 tablespoons sugar
- ¼ cup brown rice flour
- 2 tablespoons vegan butter
- ½ teaspoon ground cinnamon

**Directions:**
1. Preheat your air fryer to 350 degrees F for 5 minutes.
2. In a ramekin, combine the apple, strawberries and blueberries.
3. In a bowl, mix the rest of the ingredients.
4. Pour the mixture over the fruits and mix well.
5. Cook in the air fryer at 350 degrees F for 15 minutes.

## 100. Potato Flautas With Green Chili Sauce

Servings:2
Cooking Time: 8 Minutes Fry: 392°f
**Ingredients:**
- 1 medium potato, peeled and chopped into small cubes (1½ cups chopped potato)
- 2 tablespoons nondairy milk, plain and unsweetened
- 2 large garlic cloves, minced or pressed
- ¼ teaspoon sea salt
- ⅛ teaspoon freshly ground black pepper
- 2 tablespoons minced scallions
- 4 sprouted corn tortillas (see Ingredient Tip)
- Cooking oil spray (sunflower, safflower, or refined coconut)
- Green Chili Sauce or fresh salsa
- Guacamole or fresh avocado slices (optional)
- Cilantro, minced (optional)

**Directions:**
1. In a pot on the stovetop fitted with a steamer basket, cook the potato cubes for 15 minutes, or until tender. While they're steaming, you'll have enough time to make the Green Chili Sauce if using.
2. Transfer the cooked potato cubes to a bowl and mash with a fork or potato masher. Add the milk, garlic, salt, and pepper and stir well. Add the scallions

and stir them into the mixture. Set the bowl aside.

3. Next, warm the tortillas (so they don't break): Run them under water for a second, and then place them in an oil-sprayed air fryer basket (stacking them is fine). Fry for 1 minute.
4. Transfer the tortillas to a flat surface, laying them out individually. Place an equal amount of the potato filling in the center of each tortilla. Roll the tortilla sides up over the filling and place seam-side down in the air fryer basket (this helps prevent the tortillas from flying open). Spray the tops with oil. Fry for 7 minutes, or until the tortillas are golden-browned and lightly crisp. Serve with sauce or salsa, and any of the additional options as desired. Enjoy immediately.

### 101. Whole-grain Corn Bread

Servings:6
Cooking Time: 25 Minutes Bake: 347°f
**Ingredients:**
- 2 tablespoons ground flaxseed
- 3 tablespoons water
- ½ cup cornmeal
- ½ cup whole-wheat pastry flour
- ⅓ cup coconut sugar
- ½ tablespoon baking powder
- ¼ teaspoon sea salt
- ¼ teaspoon baking soda
- ½ tablespoon apple cider vinegar
- ½ cup plus 1 tablespoon nondairy milk (unsweetened)
- ¼ cup neutral-flavored oil (such as sunflower, safflower, or melted refined coconut)
- Cooking oil spray (sunflower, safflower, or refined coconut)

**Directions:**
1. In a small bowl, combine the flaxseed and water. Set aside for 5 minutes, or until thick and gooey.
2. In a medium bowl, add the cornmeal, flour, sugar, baking powder, salt, and baking soda. Combine thoroughly, stirring with a whisk. Set aside.
3. Add the vinegar, milk, and oil to the flaxseed mixture and stir well.

4. Add the wet mixture to the dry mixture and stir gently, just until thoroughly combined.
5. Spray (or coat) a 6-inch round, 2-inch deep baking pan with oil. Pour the batter into it and bake for 25 minutes, or until golden-browned and a knife inserted in the center comes out clean. Cut into wedges, top with a little vegan margarine if desired.

### 102. Bell Pepper And Beans Oatmeal

Servings: 2
Cooking Time: 15 Minutes
**Ingredients:**
- 1 cup steel cut oats
- 2 tablespoons canned kidney beans, drained
- 2 red bell peppers, chopped
- 4 tablespoons coconut cream
- A pinch of sweet paprika
- Salt and black pepper to the taste
- ¼ teaspoon cumin, ground

**Directions:**
1. Heat up your air fryer at 360 degrees F, add oats, beans, bell peppers, coconut cream, paprika, salt, pepper and cumin, stir, cover and cook for 16 minutes.
2. Divide into bowls and serve for breakfast.
3. Enjoy!

# Lunch & Dinner Recipes

## 103. Easy Peasy Pizza

Servings:1
Cooking Time: 9 Minutes Bake: 347°f
**Ingredients:**
- Cooking oil spray (coconut, sunflower, or safflower)
- 1 flour tortilla, preferably sprouted or whole grain
- ¼ cup vegan pizza or marinara sauce
- ⅓ cup grated vegan mozzarella cheese or Cheesy Sauce
- Toppings of your choice

**Directions:**
1. Spray the air fryer basket with oil. Place the tortilla in the air fryer basket. If the tortilla is a little bigger than the base, no probs! Simply fold the edges up a bit to form a semblance of a "crust."
2. Pour the sauce in the center, and evenly distribute it around the tortilla "crust" (I like to use the back of a spoon for this purpose).
3. Sprinkle evenly with vegan cheese, and add your toppings. Bake for 9 minutes, or until nicely browned. Remove carefully, cut into four pieces, and enjoy.

## 104. Potato And Carrot Stew

Servings: 4
Cooking Time: 25 Minutes
**Ingredients:**
- 2 carrots, chopped
- 6 potatoes, chopped
- Salt and black pepper to the taste
- 1 quart veggie stock
- ½ teaspoon smoked paprika
- A handful thyme, chopped
- 1 tablespoon parsley, chopped

**Directions:**
1. In your air fryer, mix carrots, potatoes, stock, salt, pepper, paprika, parsley and thyme, stir and cook at 375 degrees F for 25 minutes.
2. Divide into bowls and serve right away.
3. Enjoy!

## 105. Roasted Beans

Servings: 4
Cooking Time: 30 Minutes

**Ingredients:**
- 1 lb green beans
- 1/2 tsp onion powder
- 2 tbsp olive oil
- 3/4 tsp garlic powder
- 1/2 tsp pepper
- 1/2 tsp salt

**Directions:**
1. In a large bowl, add all ingredients and toss well.
2. Arrange green beans into the instant pot air fryer basket and place basket in the pot.
3. Seal the pot with air fryer lid and select bake mode and cook at 400 F for 25-30 minutes.
4. Serve and enjoy.

## 106. Quick Veggie Pasta

Servings: 4
Cooking Time: 4 Minutes
**Ingredients:**
- 1/2 lb pasta, uncooked
- 1/4 green onion, sliced
- 1/4 tsp red chili flakes
- 1 tsp ground ginger
- 1 tbsp garlic, minced
- 3 tbsp coconut amino
- 2 cups vegetable broth
- 1 1/2 cups baby spinach, chopped
- 1 cup frozen peas
- 8 oz mushrooms, sliced
- 2 carrots, peeled and chopped
- 1/4 tsp pepper
- 1 tsp salt

**Directions:**
1. Add all ingredients except spinach into the inner pot of instant pot duo crisp and stir well.
2. Seal the pot with pressure cooking lid and cook on high for 4 minutes.
3. Once done, allow to release pressure naturally. Remove lid.
4. Add spinach and stir well and let it sit for 5 minutes.
5. Serve and enjoy.

## 107. Black Bean-tomato Soup With Poblano Chili Rings

Servings: 6
Cooking Time: 25 Minutes
**Ingredients:**

- For the soup:
- 4 cups black beans, cooked and puréed
- 3 Roma tomatoes, coarsely chopped
- 3 cloves garlic
- 2 1/2 cups vegetable broth
- 1/2 white onion, medium-sized, coarsely chopped
- 1 to 2 tablespoons corn oil
- 1 teaspoon salt
- 1 ancho chili, stemmed and then seeded
- 1 1/2 cups water
- For the poblano chili rings:
- 1 poblano chili, cut into 1/2-inch thick rings
- 1/2 cup garbanzo or white bean aquafaba
- 1/2 cup panko breadcrumbs, divided
- 1/2 teaspoon salt, divided
- For garnishing:
- Poblano Chile Rings
- Ripe Hass avocado, chopped
- Tortilla strips or chips
- Vegan sour cream, vigorously whipped

**Directions:**
1. For the poblano chili rings:
2. Toss 1/4 cup panko breadcrumbs with 1/4 teaspoon salt in a shallow bowl. Do the same with the remaining panko breadcrumbs and salt in another shallow bowl. Set aside one of the bowls with the panko breadcrumb mixture.
3. Dredge the chili slices in the aquafaba and then coat with the breadcrumb mixture. The panko mixture will stick to the rings really well at first, but after the first half of the rings, it will begin to clump and no longer stick well. When this happens, use the second bowl of panko mixture.
4. In a single layer, arrange the coated chili slices in the air fryer basket – do not overlap. You may need to cook in batches.
5. Set the temperature to 390F and the timer for 8 to 10 minutes – shake the basket after 5 minutes – you want the chilies soft and the panko browned. Cook the next batches for about 6 to 8 minutes since the air fryer is already

hot. Serve right away topped with your soup.
6. For the soup:
7. Put the ancho chili, tomatoes, and water into a 3-quart pot and stir to combine. Turn the heat to medium heat and let simmer for about 10 minutes.
8. After 10 minutes, carefully transfer the soup to a blender. Add the onion and garlic into the blender and puree until smooth – hold down the cover of the blender with a clean kitchen towel to prevent the top from exploding. If you want a completely smooth puree, press the puree through a strainer.
9. Wipe the pot clean. Put the oil into the pot and heat on medium-high flame or heat. Return the puree to the pot and cook for around 5 minutes, stirring slowly. After 5 minutes, reduce the heat to medium. Add the pureed bean, salt, and broth. Simmer for 10 minutes, adding liquid if needed to make the soup creamy, but not too thick. Serve garnished with poblano chili rings and your preferred other garnishes.

### 108. Zucchini, Carrot And Squash Salad

Servings: 4
Cooking Time: 25 Minutes
**Ingredients:**
- 6 teaspoons olive oil
- 1 pound zucchinis, cut into half moons
- ½ pound carrots, cubed
- 1 yellow squash, cut into chunks
- Salt and white pepper to the taste
- 1 tablespoon tarragon, chopped
- 2 tablespoons tomato paste

**Directions:**
1. In your air fryer's pan, mix oil with zucchinis, carrots, squash, salt, pepper, tarragon and tomato paste, cover and cook at 400 degrees F for 25 minutes.
2. Divide between plates and serve.
3. Enjoy!

### 109. Spicy Thai Totchos

Servings:4
Cooking Time:15 Minutes
**Ingredients:**
- 1¼ cups Sweet Potato Tater Tots
- ½ cup bean sprouts
- ½ cup edamame beans

- ½ avocado
- 1 tablespoon sour cream (vegan / dairy free)
- 2-3 tablespoons spicy coconut almond sauce
- 1 green onion, chopped
- ½ lime, sliced

**Directions:**
1. Prepare air fryer if using. Set temp to 400 °F, cook tater tots for 7 minutes. Remove, shake to turn tater tots, add edamame. Return to air fryer and cook another 5 minutes, until tots are completely cooked through and edamame is hot.
2. Preheat oven to 425 °F if using oven. Line baking sheet with parchment.
3. On a prepared baking sheet, arrange tater tots in a single layer. Bake for 15 minutes, remove from oven.
4. Reduce oven temperature to 375 °F. Using a spatula, flip tater tots and keeping in single layer, move to one side of baking sheet. Add edamame beans in a single layer on the baking sheet, return to oven for 10 minutes more.
5. While tater tots and edamame bake, slice avocado, green onion and lime. Prepare spicy coconut almond sauce.
6. Assemble totchos: on two plates, pile tots, bean sprouts and edamame beans. Top with avocado slices, sour cream, green onion and drizzle spicy sauce and lime.

### 110. Falafel Balls

Servings: 3
Cooking Time: 12 Minutes
**Ingredients:**
- 1 can (15 ounces) chickpeas, drained and then rinsed, OR 2 cups cooked chickpeas
- 1 cup rolled oats
- 1 lemon, freshly squeezed juice only
- 1 tablespoon flax meal
- 1 teaspoon garlic powder
- 1 teaspoon ground cumin
- 1/2 cup diced sweet onion
- 1/2 cup minced carrots
- 1/2 cup roasted salted cashews
- 1/2 teaspoon turmeric

- 2 tablespoons olive oil
- 2 tablespoons soy sauce

**Directions:**
1. Put the olive oil into a large-sized frying pan and heat over medium-high heat. When the oil is hot, add the carrots and onions, and sauté for about 7 minutes or until softened. Transfer to a large-sized bowl.
2. Put the oats and cashews into a food processor. Process until the mixture resembles a coarse meal. Add the oat mixture to the bowl with the carrot mixture. Put the chickpeas into the food processor. Add the lemon juice and soy sauce and the puree until the mixture is semi-smooth – chunks are alright. You may need to stop and scrape the sides a couple of times to get the ingredients moving. Transfer the chickpea mixture to the bowl with the mixture of oat and carrot.
3. Add the spices and the flaxseed to the bowl. Using a fork, mix everything until well combined, mashing any large pieces of chickpeas in the process.
4. With clean hands, divide the mixture into 12 portions and form the portions into balls. In a single layer, arrange the balls in the air fryer basket.
5. Set the temperature to 370F and the timer for 12 minutes – shake the basket after 8 minutes.
6. Serve as desired – stuffed into pitas together with tahini dressing or serve with your preferred accompaniments.

### 111. Creole Seasoned Vegetables

Servings: 5
Cooking Time: 15 Minutes
**Ingredients:**
- ¼ cup honey
- ¼ cup yellow mustard
- 1 large red bell pepper, sliced
- 1 teaspoon black pepper
- 1 teaspoon salt
- 2 large yellow squash, cut into ½ inch thick slices
- 2 medium zucchinis, cut into ½ inch thick slices
- 2 teaspoons creole seasoning
- 2 teaspoons smoked paprika

- 3 tablespoons olive oil
- Direction:
- Preheat the air fryer to 330° F.
- Place the grill pan accessory in the air fryer.
- In a Ziploc bag, put the zucchini, squash, red bell pepper, olive oil, salt and pepper. Give a shake to season all vegetables.
- Place on the grill pan and cook for 15 minutes.
- Meanwhile, prepare the sauce by combining the mustard, honey, paprika, and creole seasoning. Season with salt to taste.
- Serve the vegetables with the sauce.

### 112. Sweetcorn Risotto

Servings: 4
Cooking Time: 13 Minutes
**Ingredients:**
- 1 cup Arborio rice
- 1/2 cup sweet corn
- 1 tsp mix herbs
- 3 cups vegetable stock
- 1 tbsp olive oil
- 1 tsp garlic, minced
- 1/2 cup peas
- 1 red pepper, diced
- 1 large onion, chopped
- 1/4 pepper
- 1/2 tsp salt

**Directions:**
1. Add oil into the inner pot of instant pot duo crisp and set pot on sauté mode.
2. Add onion and garlic and sauté for 5 minutes.
3. Add rice and stir to combine.
4. Add remaining ingredients and stir well.
5. Seal the pot with pressure cooking lid and cook on high for 8 minutes.
6. Once done, release pressure using a quick release. Remove lid.
7. Serve and enjoy.

### 113. Eggplant Stew With Herbed Okra

Servings: 10
Cooking Time: 25 Minutes
**Ingredients:**
- 2 cups eggplant, cubed
- 1 butternut squash, peeled and cubed

- 2 cups zucchini, cubed
- 10 ounces tomato sauce
- 1 carrot, sliced
- 1 yellow onion, chopped
- ½ cup veggie stock
- 10 ounces okra
- 1/3 cup raisins
- 2 garlic cloves, minced
- ½ teaspoon turmeric powder
- ½ teaspoon cumin, ground
- ½ teaspoon red pepper flakes, crushed
- ¼ teaspoon sweet paprika
- ¼ teaspoon cinnamon powder

**Directions:**
1. In your air fryer, mix eggplant with squash, zucchini, tomato sauce, carrot, onion, okra, garlic, stock, raisins, turmeric, cumin, pepper flakes, paprika and cinnamon, stir, cover and cook at 360 degrees F for 25 minutes.
2. Divide into bowls and serve.
3. Enjoy!

### 114. Cheesy Potato Gratin

Servings: 6
Cooking Time: 30 Minutes
**Ingredients:**
- 3 medium potatoes, sliced 1/8-inch thick
- 3 cups cheddar cheese, shredded
- 3/4 cup heavy cream
- 3/4 tsp garlic powder
- 1 tbsp butter
- 1/4 tsp pepper
- 1/2 tsp sea salt

**Directions:**
1. Spray 8-inch round pan with cooking spray.
2. Layer the sliced potatoes in prepared pan.
3. Season each layer with garlic powder, pepper, and salt then pour 1 tablespoon of heavy cream over potato layer and sprinkle thin layer of shredded cheese.
4. Layer sliced potatoes until you have 5 layers.
5. Top with remaining cream and cheese.
6. Pour 1 1/2 cups of water into the instant pot duo crisp then place the trivet in the pot.
7. Place pan on top of the trivet.

8. Seal the pot with pressure cooking lid and cook on pressure cook mode for 25 minutes.
9. Once done, release pressure using a quick release. Remove lid.
10. Seal the pot with air fryer lid and select broil mode for 5 minutes.
11. Once done then remove the pan from instant pot and let it cool for 10 minutes.
12. Serve and enjoy.

## 115. Buttery Carrots With Pancetta

Servings: 5
Cooking Time: 20 Minutes
**Ingredients:**
- 4 oz. pancetta, diced
- 1 medium leek, white and pale green parts only, sliced lengthwise, washed and thinly sliced
- 1/4 cup moderately sweet white wine (I used dry Riesling)
- 1 pound baby carrots
- 1/2 tsp. ground black pepper
- 2 tbsp. unsalted butter, cut into small bits

**Directions:**
1. Put the pancetta in the Ninja Foodi turned to the Air Crisp function.
2. Use time adjustment button to set cooking time to 5 minutes.
3. Add the leeks; cook, often stirring, until softened.
4. Pour in the wine and scrape up any browned bits at the bottom of the pot as it comes to a simmer.
5. Add the carrots and pepper; stir well.
6. Scrape and pour the contents of the Ninja Foodi Multicooker into a 1-quart, round, high-sided soufflé or baking dish. Dot with the bits of butter.
7. Lay a piece of parchment paper on top of the dish, then a piece of aluminum foil.
8. Seal the foil tightly over the baking dish.
9. Set the Ninja Foodi Multicooker rack inside, and pour in 2 cups water.
10. Use aluminum foil to build a sling for the baking dish; lower the baking dish into the cooker.
11. Lock the lid on the Ninja Foodi Multicooker and then cook for 7 minutes. To get 7-minutes cook time,

press "Pressure" button and use the Time Adjustment button to adjust the cook time to 7 minutes.
12. Use the quick-release method to return the pot's pressure to normal.
13. Close the crisping lid. Select BROIL, and set the time to 5 minutes.
14. Select START/StoP to begin. Cook until top has browned.
15. Unlock and open the pot. Use the foil sling to lift the baking dish out of the cooker.
16. Uncover and stir well. Serve and enjoy!

## 116. Healthy Roasted Vegetables

Servings： 4
Cooking Time: 45 Minutes
**Ingredients:**
- 2 potatoes, cut into chunks
- 3 medium carrots, peeled and cut into chunks
- 1 small rutabaga, peeled and cut into chunks
- 2 parsnips, peeled and cut into chunks
- 1/4 cup olive oil
- Pepper
- Salt

**Directions:**
1. In a large bowl, toss vegetable with oil.
2. Transfer vegetables into the instant pot air fryer basket and season with pepper and salt.
3. Place air fryer basket in the pot.
4. Seal the pot with air fryer lid and select roast mode and cook at 400 F for 35-45 minutes.

## 117. Sweet Potato And Beans Burger

Servings： 4
Cooking Time: 12 Minutes
**Ingredients:**
- 1 cup canned black beans, drained and rinsed
- 2 cups mashed sweet potatoes
- 1 cup cooked quinoa
- Salt and black pepper to taste
- ½ cup almond meal
- 1 tsp smoked paprika
- ½ cup chopped green onion
- To assemble:
- 4 buns, halved
- 4 lettuce leaves

- 4 slices tomatoes

**Directions:**

1. Mash half of the black beans in a medium bowl and combine with the remaining patties ingredients including the whole beans. Mold four cakes out of the mixture. If too soft, mix with 1 to 2 tablespoons more of almond meal.
2. Preheat the air fryer and place 2 patties in the fryer basket. Oil lightly with cooking spray and bake at 390 F for 12 minutes. Flip after 7 minutes.
3. Remove onto a plate and bake the remaining.
4. To assemble, line four bottom halves of each bun with lettuce leaves, place a patty on each and top with a slice of tomato each. Cover with the other bun halves and serve immediately.

### 118. Creamy 'n Cheese Broccoli Bake

Servings: 2
Cooking Time: 30 Minutes

**Ingredients:**

- 1-pound fresh broccoli, coarsely chopped
- 2 tablespoons all-purpose flour
- salt to taste
- 1 tablespoon dry bread crumbs, or to taste
- 1/2 large onion, coarsely chopped
- 1/2 (14 ounce) can evaporated milk, divided
- 1/2 cup cubed sharp Cheddar cheese
- 1-1/2 teaspoons butter, or to taste
- 1/4 cup water
- Direction:
- Lightly grease baking pan of air fryer with cooking spray. Mix in half of the milk and flour in pan and for 5 minutes, cook on 360° F. Halfway through cooking time, mix well. Add broccoli and remaining milk. Mix well and cook for another 5 minutes.
- Stir in cheese and mix well until melted.
- In a small bowl mix well, butter and bread crumbs. Sprinkle on top of broccoli.
- Cook for 20 minutes at 360° F until tops are lightly browned.
- Serve and enjoy.

### 119. Healthy Quinoa Black Bean Chili

Servings: 6
Cooking Time: 12 Minutes

**Ingredients:**

- 1/2 cup quinoa, rinsed and drained
- 14 oz can black beans, rinsed and drained
- 14 oz can tomato, diced
- 2 tbsp tomato paste
- 4 cups vegetable broth
- 2 celery stalks, diced
- 1 tsp garlic, minced
- 1 onion, chopped
- 1 tsp chili powder
- 1 tsp ground coriander
- 2 tsp ground cumin
- 2 tsp paprika
- 3 sweet potatoes, peeled and diced
- 1 bell pepper, diced
- 1 tsp salt

**Directions:**

1. Add all ingredients into the inner pot of instant pot duo crisp and stir well.
2. Seal the pot with pressure cooking lid and cook on high for 12 minutes.
3. Once done, release pressure using a quick release. Remove lid.
4. Stir and serve.

### 120. Eggplant And Tomato Sauce

Servings: 2
Cooking Time: 12 Minutes

**Ingredients:**

- 4 cups eggplant, cubed
- 1 tablespoon olive oil
- 1 tablespoon garlic powder
- A pinch of salt and black pepper
- 3 garlic cloves, minced
- 1 cup tomato sauce

**Directions:**

1. In a pan that fits your air fryer, combine eggplant cubes with oil, garlic, salt, pepper, garlic powder and tomato sauce, toss, place in your air fryer and cook at 370 degrees F for 12 minutes.
2. Divide between plates and serve.
3. Enjoy!

### 121. Spicy Veggie Recipe From Thailand

Servings: 4
Cooking Time: 15 Minutes

**Ingredients:**
- 1 ½ cups packed cilantro leaves
- 1 tablespoon black pepper
- 1 tablespoon chili garlic sauce
- 1/3 cup vegetable oil
- 2 pounds vegetable of your choice, sliced into cubes
- 2 tablespoons fish sauce
- 8 cloves of garlic, minced
- Direction:
- Preheat the air fryer to 330° F.
- Place the grill pan accessory in the air fryer.
- Place all
- Put in the grill pan and cook for 15 minutes.

### 122. Veggie Risotto

Servings:   4
Cooking Time: 13 Minutes
**Ingredients:**
- 1 cup Arborio rice
- 1/2 cup peas
- 1 red pepper, diced
- 1 onion, chopped
- 1 tsp dried mix herbs
- 3 cups vegetable stock
- 1 tbsp olive oil
- 1 tsp garlic, minced
- 1/2 cup corn
- 1/4 pepper
- 1/2 tsp salt

**Directions:**
1. Add oil into the inner pot of instant pot duo crisp and set pot on sauté mode.
2. Add onion and garlic and sauté for 5 minutes.
3. Add rice and stir well. Add remaining ingredients and stir well.
4. Seal the pot with pressure cooking lid and cook on high for 8 minutes.
5. Once done, release pressure using a quick release. Remove lid.
6. Stir and serve.

### 123. Easy Broccoli Mix

Servings: 4
Cooking Time: 20 Minutes
**Ingredients:**
- 2 broccoli heads, florets separated
- Juice of ½ lemon

- 1 tablespoon olive oil
- 2 teaspoons sweet paprika
- Salt and black pepper to the taste
- 3 garlic cloves, minced
- 1 tablespoon sesame seeds

**Directions:**
1. In a bowl, mix broccoli with lemon juice, olive oil, paprika, salt, pepper and garlic, toss to coat, transfer to your air fryer's basket, cook at 360 degrees G for 15 minutes, sprinkle sesame seeds, cook for 5 minutes more and divide between plates.
2. Serve right away.
3. Enjoy!

### 124. White Beans With Rosemary

Servings: 10
Cooking Time: 20 Minutes
**Ingredients:**
- 2 pounds white beans, cooked
- 3 celery stalks, chopped
- 2 carrots, chopped
- 1 bay leaf
- 1 yellow onion, chopped
- 3 garlic cloves, minced
- 1 teaspoon rosemary, dried
- 1 teaspoon oregano, dried
- 1 teaspoon thyme, dried
- A drizzle of olive oil
- Salt and black pepper to the taste
- 28 ounces canned tomatoes, chopped
- 6 cups chard, chopped

**Directions:**
1. In your air fryer's pan, mix white beans with celery, carrots, bay leaf, onion, garlic, rosemary, oregano, thyme, oil, salt, pepper, tomatoes and chard, toss, cover and cook at 365 degrees F for 20 minutes.
2. Divide into bowls and serve.
3. Enjoy!

### 125. Mushroom & Green Bean Casserole

Servings: 6
Cooking Time: 10 Minutes
**Ingredients:**
- 24 oz. green beans, trimmed
- 2 cups button mushrooms, sliced
- 1 tablespoon lemon juice
- 1 tablespoon garlic powder

- ¾ teaspoon ground sage
- 1 teaspoon onion powder
- Salt and pepper to taste
- Cooking spray

**Directions:**
1. Combine all the ingredients in a bowl.
2. Transfer to the air fryer basket and coat with oil.
3. Cook at 400 degrees F for 12 minutes.
4. Shake every 3 minutes.

### 126. Artichoke Pesto Pasta With Air Fried Chickpeas

Servings:4
Cooking Time:15 Minutes
**Ingredients:**
- 8 ounces vegan pappardelle or other pasta
- 1 packed cup (1 ounce) fresh basil leaves
- 6 jarred artichoke hearts, drained and squeezed slightly to remove excess liquid
- 2 Tablespoons shelled pumpkin seeds (pepitas)
- Juice of half a lemon (~1 Tablespoon)
- 1 clove garlic
- ½ teaspoon white miso paste
- 1 teaspoon extra virgin olive oil (optional)
- 1 batch air-fried or roasted chickpeas

**Directions:**
1. Cook pasta according to package Directions:.
2. While pasta is cooking, combine basil leaves, artichoke hearts, shelled pumpkin seeds, lemon juice, garlic, and white miso paste in a food processor until it is fully combined. Scrape down the sides, as needed, and continue processing until the pesto is mostly smooth.
3. After the pasta is finished cooking, drain in a colander.
4. Move the noodles to a large mixing bowl, and toss with extra virgin olive oil to prevent sticking (optional). Spoon the artichoke pesto over the pasta, and toss until evenly combined.
5. Serve pasta topped with air fried or roasted chickpeas.

### 127. Lemon Tofu

Servings: 4
Cooking Time: 25 Minutes
**Ingredients:**
- 1 lb. tofu, sliced into cubes
- 1 tablespoon tamari
- 1 tablespoon arrowroot powder
- ¼ cup lemon juice
- 1 teaspoon lemon zest
- 2 tablespoon sugar
- ½ cup water
- aspoons cornstarch

**Directions:**
1. Coat the tofu cubes in tamari.
2. Dredge with arrowroot powder.
3. Let sit for 15 minutes.
4. Add the rest of the ingredients in a bowl, mix and set aside.
5. Cook the tofu in the air fryer at 390 degrees F for 10 minutes, shaking halfway through.
6. Put the tofu in a skillet over medium high heat.
7. Stir in the sauce.
8. Simmer until the sauce has thickened.
9. Serve with rice or vegetables.

### 128. Chickpea Tacos

Servings: 4
Cooking Time: 20 Minutes
**Ingredients:**
- 19 oz. canned chickpeas, rinsed and drained
- 4 cups cauliflower florets, chopped
- 2 tablespoons olive oil
- 2 tablespoons taco seasoning
- 4 tortillas
- 4 cups cabbage, shredded
- 2 avocados, sliced
- Soy yogurt

**Directions:**
1. Preheat your air fryer to 390 degrees F.
2. Toss the chickpeas and cauliflower in olive oil.
3. Sprinkle with taco seasoning.
4. Put in the air fryer basket.
5. Cook for 20 minutes, shaking occasionally.
6. Stuff filling into the tortillas and top with cabbage, avocado and yogurt.

## 129. Baked Beans

Servings: 4
Cooking Time: 40 Minutes
**Ingredients:**

- 1 cup navy beans, dry, soaked overnight and drained
- 2 tbsp tomato paste
- 1/2 tbsp vinegar
- 1/2 tbsp Worcestershire sauce
- 1/2 tsp mustard
- 1 onion, chopped
- 1 tbsp olive oil
- 1/2 cup water
- 1/2 cup vegetable stock
- 1 1/2 tbsp molasses
- 2 tbsp brown sugar
- 1/2 tsp pepper
- 1/2 tsp sea salt

**Directions:**

1. Add oil into the inner pot of instant pot duo crisp and set pot on sauté mode.
2. Add onion and sauté for 3 minutes.
3. Add remaining ingredients and stir to combine.
4. Seal the pot with pressure cooking lid and cook on high for 40 minutes.
5. Once done, release pressure using a quick release. Remove lid.
6. Stir well and serve.

## 130. Simple Veggie Salad

Servings: 8
Cooking Time: 10 Minutes
**Ingredients:**

- 1 and ½ cups tomatoes, chopped
- 3 cups eggplant, chopped
- 2 teaspoons capers
- Cooking spray
- 3 garlic cloves, minced
- 2 teaspoons balsamic vinegar
- 1 tablespoon basil, chopped
- A pinch of salt and black pepper

**Directions:**

1. Grease a pan that fits your air fryer with cooking spray, add tomatoes, eggplant, capers, garlic, salt and pepper, place in your air fryer and cook at 365 degrees F for 10 minutes.
2. Divide between plates, drizzle balsamic vinegar all over, sprinkle basil and serve cold.

3. Enjoy!

## 131. Smoky Sweet Crunchy Chickpeas

Servings:4
Cooking Time:10 Minutes
**Ingredients:**

- 1 (15 ounce) can chickpeas
- 2 tablespoons aquafaba from chickpeas
- 1 tablespoon maple syrup
- 2 teaspoons smoked paprika
- 1½ teaspoons garlic powder
- ½ teaspoon sea salt

**Directions:**

1. Drain chickpeas, reserving aquafaba. Do not rinse chickpeas.
2. Add chickpeas to air fryer basket, shake to a single layer, place inside air fryer. Fry at 390 °F for 8 minutes.
3. While the chickpeas cook: in mixing bowl, whisk together 2 tablespoons aquafaba, maple syrup, smoked paprika, garlic powder, and salt. (Save the remaining aquafaba for another use.)
4. Add chickpeas fresh from air fryer, stir to coat completely. Return flavored chickpeas to air fryer basket, using a spatula to get every last bit of the sauce.
5. Return chickpeas to air fryer. Fry at 390 °F for another 5 minutes. Shake basket, return to fryer for another 3-5 minutes, until chickpeas are crisp.
6. Transfer to serving bowl. Serve warm or room temperature - as a party appetizer, salad topper, or snack!
7. (These chickpeas can also be roasted in the oven.)

## 132. Red Bean-chipotle Burgers

Servings:4
Cooking Time:10 Minutes
**Ingredients:**

- 1 small onion , peeled and cut into quarters
- 1 clove garlic
- 1 16-ounce can kidney beans , drained and rinsed
- ½ cup old fashioned or quick oats , uncooked
- ½ cup cooked brown rice

- 1-3 teaspoons chopped canned chipotles OR ½-2 teaspoons chipotle chile powder or hot smoked paprika, to taste
- 2 tablespoons whole wheat flour or brown rice flour (or other flour)
- 1 tablespoon tomato paste
- ½ teaspoon salt (optional for salt-free diets)
- ½ teaspoon oregano
- ½ teaspoon thyme

**Directions:**
1. Preheat air fryer to 390F. Form burgers on parchment paper and transfer to air fryer (I put them directly into the AF but they did stick; if possible, cut parchment paper to fit AF.) Cook for 8 minutes.
2. Turn burgers over and rearrange from top to bottom if you are using a rack. Cook 4-8 more minutes, until burgers are crispy outside and firm. Be careful not to overcook or they will be hard.

### 133. Pepper-pineapple With Butter-sugar Glaze

Servings: 2
Cooking Time: 10 Minutes
**Ingredients:**
- 1 medium-sized pineapple, peeled and sliced
- 1 red bell pepper, seeded and julienned
- 1 teaspoon brown sugar
- 2 teaspoons melted butter
- Salt to taste
- Direction:
- Preheat the air fryer to 390° F.
- Place the grill pan accessory in the air fryer.
- Mix all ingredients in a Ziploc bag and give a good shake.
- Dump onto the grill pan and cook for 10 minutes making sure that you flip the pineapples every 5 minutes.

### 134. Chickpea Cauliflower Tacos

Servings: 2
Cooking Time: 20 Minutes
**Ingredients:**
- 1 tsp Mexican seasoning
- 1 (15 oz) can chickpea, drained and rinsed

- 2 cups cauliflower florets
- Salt and freshly ground black pepper to taste
- 4 corn tortillas
- 1 cup shredded red cabbage
- 1 avocado, pitted and sliced
- 1 jalapeno, sliced and seeded
- Dairy free sour cream for topping

**Directions:**
1. Mix the Mexican seasoning with the chickpeas, cauliflower, salt, and black pepper.
2. Preheat the air fryer and spoon the chickpeas and cauliflower into the fryer basket. Roast at 350 F for 20 minutes, shaking the basket halfway.
3. When ready, spoon the mixture into a bowl and assemble the tacos.
4. Share the chickpeas and cauliflower into the corn tortillas. Top with the cabbage, jalapeno, and avocado.
5. Drizzle the sour cream on top and serve immediately.

### 135. Lemony Endive Mix

Servings: 4
Cooking Time: 10 Minutes
**Ingredients:**
- 8 endives, trimmed
- Salt and black pepper to the taste
- 3 tablespoons olive oil
- Juice of ½ lemon
- 1 tablespoon tomato paste
- 2 tablespoons parsley, chopped
- 1 teaspoon stevia

**Directions:**
1. In a bowl, combine endives with salt, pepper, oil, lemon juice, tomato paste, parsley and stevia, toss, place endives in your air fryer's basket and cook at 365 degrees F for 10 minutes.
2. Divide between plates and serve.
3. Enjoy!

### 136. Delicious Chickpea Hummus

Servings: 10
Cooking Time: 45 Minutes
**Ingredients:**
- 1 cup chickpeas, dried
- 3 garlic cloves, minced
- 3 cups vegetable broth
- 1 tbsp fresh lemon juice

- 2 tbsp olive oil
- 1 tsp salt

**Directions:**
1. Add broth, chickpeas, and salt into the inner pot of instant pot duo crisp.
2. Seal the pot with pressure cooking lid and high for 45 minutes.
3. Once done, release pressure using a quick release. Remove lid.
4. Drain chickpeas well and transfer to the food processor along with remaining ingredients and process until smooth.
5. Serve and enjoy.

### 137. Crispy Cauliflower Bites

Servings: 4
Cooking Time: 12 Minutes
**Ingredients:**
- 3 garlic cloves, minced
- 1 tbsp. olive oil
- 1/2 tsp. salt
- 1/2 tsp. smoked paprika
- 4 cups cauliflower florets

**Directions:**
1. Place in the ceramic pot the Foodi Cook and Crisp basket.
2. Place all ingredients in a bowl and toss to combine.
3. Place the seasoned cauliflower florets in the basket.
4. Close the crisping lid and press the Air Crisp button before pressing the START button.
5. Adjust the cooking time to 10 minutes.
6. Give the basket a shake while cooking for even cooking. Serve and enjoy!

### 138. Mixed Vegetable Bowls

Servings： 4
Cooking Time: 1 Hour 10 Minutes
**Ingredients:**
- 1 cup cauliflower florets
- 1 cup broccoli florets
- 1 small zucchini, chopped
- 2 tbsp garlic-ginger puree
- 1 tbsp onion powder
- 2 tbsp olive oil
- 1 tbsp curry paste
- 2 tsp mixed spice
- 1 ½ cups coconut milk
- Salt and freshly ground black pepper as needed

**Directions:**
1. In a medium bowl, combine the cauliflower, broccoli, zucchini, ginger-garlic paste, onion powder, olive oil, curry paste, mixed spices, and coconut milk. Stir to be well mixed.
2. Cover the bowl with a plastic wrap and refrigerate for 1 hour to marinate the vegetables.
3. Preheat the air fryer.
4. Remove the veggies from the fridge and use a slotted spoon to fetch some vegetables into the fryer basket making sure to drip off as much liquid as possible.
5. Crisp the veggies at 350 F for 10 minutes or until softened and golden brown.
6. Spoon the vegetables into a serving bowl and serve with coconut sauce.

### 139. Crispy Honey Carrots

Servings: 2
Cooking Time: 10 Minutes
**Ingredients:**
- 3 cups carrots, cut into 1/2-inch pieces
- 1 tbsp honey
- 1 tbsp olive oil
- Pepper
- Salt

**Directions:**
1. Add carrots in a mixing bowl then add honey, oil, pepper, and salt and toss to coat.
2. Transfer carrots into the instant pot duo crisp air fryer basket then place basket in the instant pot.
3. Seal the pot with air fryer lid and air fry carrots for 10 minutes at 400 F. Toss carrots after 5 minutes.
4. Serve and enjoy.

### 140. Simple Endive Mix

Servings: 4
Cooking Time: 10 Minutes
**Ingredients:**
- 8 endives, trimmed
- Salt and black pepper to the taste
- 3 tablespoons olive oil
- Juice of ½ lemon
- 1 tablespoon tomato paste
- 2 tablespoons parsley, chopped

- 1 teaspoon stevia

**Directions:**
1. In a bowl, combine endives with salt, pepper, oil, lemon juice, tomato paste, parsley and stevia, toss, place endives in your air fryer's basket and cook at 365 degrees F for 10 minutes.
2. Divide between plates and serve.
3. Enjoy!

### 141. Mexican Casserole

Servings: 4
Cooking Time: 15 Minutes
**Ingredients:**
- 1 tablespoon olive oil
- 4 garlic cloves, minced
- 1 yellow onion, chopped
- 2 tablespoons cilantro, chopped
- 1 small red chili, chopped
- 2 teaspoons cumin, ground
- Salt and black pepper to the taste
- 1 teaspoon sweet paprika
- 1 teaspoon coriander seeds
- 1 pound sweet potatoes, cubed
- Juice of ½ lime
- 10 ounces green beans
- 2 cups tomatoes, chopped
- 1 tablespoon parsley, chopped

**Directions:**
1. Grease a pan that fits your air fryer with the oil, add garlic, onion, cilantro, red chili, cumin, salt, pepper, paprika, coriander, potatoes, lime juice, green beans and tomatoes, toss, place in your air fryer and cook at 365 degrees F for 15 minutes.
2. Add parsley, divide between plates and serve.
3. Enjoy!

### 142. Garlic Rice Stuffed Mushrooms

Servings: 4
Cooking Time: 15 Minutes
**Ingredients:**
- 1 cup cooked short grain rice
- ½ cup black beans, drained and rinsed
- 3 cloves garlic, minced
- 1 tsp coriander powder
- Salt and freshly ground black pepper
- 1 tbsp olive oil + extra for drizzling
- ½ tbsp chopped parsley

- ½ tbsp. chopped oregano
- 16 small button mushrooms cups

**Directions:**
1. In a bowl, mix all the ingredients except the mushroom caps.
2. Preheat the air fryer.
3. In each mushroom cup, spoon the rice mixture to the brim of the mushrooms.
4. Drizzle with some olive oil and place 5 to 6 mushrooms in the fryer basket.
5. Slide the basket into the air fryer and bake at 370 F for 10 to 15 minutes or until the mushrooms nicely brown.
6. Transfer to a plate when ready and cook the remaining mushrooms.
7. Garnish with extra parsley and serve warm with tomato sauce.

### 143. Fried Tofu Recipe From Malaysia

Servings: 4
Cooking Time: 30 Minutes
**Ingredients:**
- 1 block tofu, cut into strips
- 1 tablespoon maple syrup
- 1 teaspoon sriracha sauce
- 2 cloves of garlic
- 2 tablespoons soy sauce
- 2 teaspoons fresh ginger no need to peel, coarsely chopped
- juice of 1 fresh lime
- Peanut Butter Sauce
- 1 tablespoon soy sauce
- 1/2 cup creamy peanut butter
- 1-2 teaspoons Sriracha sauce to taste
- 2 cloves of garlic
- 2-inch piece of fresh ginger coarsely chopped
- 6 tablespoons of water
- juice of 1/2 a fresh lemon
- Direction:
- In a blender, blend all peanut butter sauce
- In same blender, blend garlic, sriracha, ginger, maple syrup, lime juice, and soy sauce until smooth. Pour into a bowl and add strips of tofu, Marinate for 30 minutes.
- With the steel skewer, skewer tofu strips.
- Place on skewer rack and air fry for 15 minutes at 370° F.
- Serve and enjoy.

## 144. Crispy Vegetable Fries Fries

Servings: 4
Cooking Time: 8 Minutes
**Ingredients:**
- 1 cup of panko breadcrumbs (regular or gluten-free)
- 1 cup rice flour
- 2 tablespoons Vegan Egg powder (I used Follow Your Heart)
- 2 tablespoons nutritional yeast flakes, divided
- 2/3 cup cold water
- Assorted vegetables of your choice, sliced into shapes similar to French fry or into bite-size chunks (such as green beans, cauliflower, zucchini, sweet onions, or squash)
- Salt and pepper

**Directions:**
1. Prepare 3 pieces of shallow dishes on a counter. Put rice flour in 1 of the dish. In the second dish, whisk the egg powder with 2/3 cup water and 1 tablespoon nutritional yeast until the mixture is smooth. In the third dish, mix the panko breadcrumbs with the remaining 1 tablespoon nutritional yeast and then add a couple pinches pepper and salt.
2. Working 1 vegetable piece at a time, coat with rice flour, into the vegan egg mixture, and finally in the breadcrumb mix, pressing to set the coating. Prepare as many veggies as you desire.
3. Lightly spritz the air fryer with oil. Alternatively, you can line the air fryer basket with parchment paper that is smaller than the basket. Carefully put the coated veggies in the air fryer basket and gently spritz with oil. Set the temperature to 380F and the timer for 8 minutes. Cook for additional minutes, if needed.
4. Serve while still crispy and hot with your choice of dipping sauce.

## 145. Fried Sweet Potato And Homemade Guacamole

Servings: 2
Cooking Time: 30 Minutes
**Ingredients:**
- For the fries:
- 1-2 sweet potatoes, medium-sized, washed and peel left on
- 1 tablespoon of coconut oil, melted
- For the guacamole:
- 1 bunch of fresh herbs, roughly chopped, I used rosemary, oregano, and parsley
- 1 ripe avocado, large-sized
- 1 sized cucumber, medium-sized, sliced and diced
- 1 sized tomato, medium-sized, sliced and diced
- 1 teaspoon garlic powder
- Himalayan Pink Salt, to taste
- Pepper, to taste

**Directions:**
1. For the fries:
2. Slice the sweet potatoes lengthwise into long-shaped pieces and then put them in a mixing bowl. Add the coconut oil and toss to coat.
3. Put into the air fryer basket. Set the temperature to 375F or 190C and set the timer for 20-30 minutes or until cooked and golden – shake halfway through cooking.
4. When the fries are cooked, transfer to a serving platter or serving bowl and sprinkle with additional salt. Serve with the guacamole.
5. For the guacamole:
6. While the sweet potato fries are baking, prepare all the ingredients as described above.
7. Slice the avocado into halves; discard the seeds and pith. Put the avocado meat in a mixing bowl and mash to desired consistency.
8. Add the rest of the ingredients and stir to combine. Refrigerate until the fries are cooked.

## 146. Easy Dill Carrots

Servings: 4
Cooking Time: 2 Hours
**Ingredients:**
- 1 lb carrots, cut round slices
- 1/2 tsp butter
- 3/4 tbsp fresh dill, minced
- 3 tbsp water

**Directions:**
1. Add all ingredients into the inner pot of instant pot duo crisp and stir well.

2. Seal the pot with pressure cooking lid and select slow cook mode and cook on low for 2 hours.
3. Stir and serve.

## 147. Sweet & Spicy Cauliflower

Servings: 4
Cooking Time: 30 Minutes
**Ingredients:**
- 4 cups cauliflower florets
- 1 onion, chopped
- 5 cloves garlic, chopped
- 1 ½ tablespoons tamari
- 1 tablespoon rice vinegar
- ½ teaspoon coconut sugar
- 1 tablespoon hot sauce
- 2 scallions, chopped

**Directions:**
1. Put the cauliflower in the air fryer basket.
2. Cook at 350 degrees F for 10 minutes, shaking halfway through.
3. Add the onion and cook for another 10 minutes.
4. Add the garlic and stir.
5. Cook for 5 more minutes.
6. In a bowl, mix all the ingredients except the scallions.
7. Add to the air fryer. Mix well.
8. Cook for 5 minutes.
9. Sprinkle scallions on top before serving.

## 148. Spicy Rice

Servings: 2
Cooking Time: 3 Minutes
**Ingredients:**
- 1 cup rice, long grain
- 1/4 cup green hot sauce
- 1/2 cup fresh cilantro, chopped
- 1/2 avocado flesh
- 1 1/4 cup vegetable broth
- Pepper
- Salt

**Directions:**
1. Add broth and rice in the inner pot of instant pot duo crisp and stir well.
2. Seal the pot with pressure cooking lid and cook on high for 3 minutes.
3. Once done, allow to release pressure naturally. Remove lid.
4. Fluff the rice using a fork.

5. Add green sauce, avocado and cilantro in a blender and blend until smooth.
6. Pour blended mixture into the rice and stir well to combine. Season with pepper and salt.
7. Serve and enjoy.

## 149. Cheddar, Squash 'n Zucchini Casserole

Servings: 4
Cooking Time: 30 Minutes
**Ingredients:**
- 1 egg
- 5 saltine crackers, or as needed, crushed
- 2 tablespoons bread crumbs
- 1/2-pound yellow squash, sliced
- 1/2-pound zucchini, sliced
- 1/2 cup shredded Cheddar cheese
- 1-1/2 teaspoons white sugar
- 1/2 teaspoon salt
- 1/4 onion, diced
- 1/4 cup biscuit baking mix
- 1/4 cup butter
- Direction:
- Lightly grease baking pan of air fryer with cooking spray. Add onion, zucchini, and yellow squash. Cover pan with foil and for 15 minutes, cook on 360° F or until tender.
- Stir in salt, sugar, egg, butter, baking mix, and cheddar cheese. Mix well. Fold in crushed crackers. Top with bread crumbs.
- Cook for 15 minutes at 390° F until tops are lightly browned.
- Serve and enjoy.

## 150. Eggplant Parmigiana

Servings: 4
Cooking Time: 40 Minutes Fry: 392°f
**Ingredients:**
- 1 medium eggplant (about 1 pound), sliced into ½-inch-thick rounds
- 2 tablespoons tamari or shoyu
- 3 tablespoons nondairy milk, plain and unsweetened
- 1 cup chickpea flour (see Substitution Tip)
- 1 tablespoon dried basil
- 1 tablespoon dried oregano
- 2 teaspoons garlic granules
- 2 teaspoons onion granules

- ½ teaspoon sea salt
- ½ teaspoon freshly ground black pepper
- Cooking oil spray (sunflower, safflower, or refined coconut)
- Vegan marinara sauce (your choice)
- Shredded vegan cheese (preferably mozzarella; see Ingredient Tip)

**Directions:**
1. Place the eggplant slices in a large bowl, and pour the tamari and milk over the top. Turn the pieces over to coat them as evenly as possible with the liquids. Set aside.
2. Make the coating: In a medium bowl, combine the flour, basil, oregano, garlic, onion, salt, and pepper and stir well. Set aside.
3. Spray the air fryer basket with oil and set aside.
4. Stir the eggplant slices again and transfer them to a plate (stacking is fine). Do not discard the liquid in the bowl.
5. Bread the eggplant by tossing an eggplant round in the flour mixture. Then, dip in the liquid again. Double up on the coating by placing the eggplant again in the flour mixture, making sure that all sides are nicely breaded. Place in the air fryer basket.
6. Repeat with enough eggplant rounds to make a (mostly) single layer in the air fryer basket. (You'll need to cook it in batches, so that you don't have too much overlap and it cooks perfectly.)
7. Spray the tops of the eggplant with enough oil so that you no longer see dry patches in the coating. Fry for 8 minutes. Remove the air fryer basket and spray the tops again. Turn each piece over, again taking care not to overlap the rounds too much. Spray the tops with oil, again making sure that no dry patches remain. Fry for another 8 minutes, or until nicely browned and crisp.
8. Repeat steps 5 to 7 one more time, or until all of the eggplant is crisp and browned.
9. Finally, place half of the eggplant in a 6-inch round, 2-inch deep baking pan and top with marinara sauce and a sprinkle of vegan cheese. Fry for 3 minutes, or until the sauce is hot and cheese is melted (be careful not to overcook, or the eggplant edges will burn). Serve immediately, plain or over pasta. Otherwise, you can store the eggplant in the fridge for several days and then make a fresh batch whenever the mood strikes by repeating this step!

### 151. Oil-free Vegan Samosa

Servings: 2-4
Cooking Time: 6 Minutes
**Ingredients:**
- For the potato filling:
- 1 clove garlic, crushed
- 1 onion, small-sized, finely chopped
- 1 potato, medium-sized, peeled and then mashed
- 1 teaspoon cumin powder
- 1 teaspoon ground coriander
- 1/2 cup carrots and pea mixture - frozen is okay
- 1/2-1 teaspoon curry powder
- 1/4 teaspoon turmeric powder
- 2 teaspoons organic coconut oil
- Sea salt, to taste
- Black pepper, to taste
- For the cheese filling:
- 4 sheets rice paper
- 2 tablespoons Tofutti cream cheese
- 2 tablespoons parsley, finely chopped
- 1 teaspoon lemon juice
- 1 teaspoon extra virgin olive oil
- 1 tablespoon nutritional yeast
- 1 serving (3 ounces) firm tofu
- Black pepper, to taste
- Sea salt, to taste
- Chili powder, to taste, optional

**Directions:**
1. Put the coconut oil in a medium-sized pot and heat. When the oil is hot, add the coriander, cumin, curry powder, and onion, and then sauté until translucent.
2. Add the carrots and peas, and then stir over medium heat for a couple of minutes.
3. Add the mashed potato and turmeric. Season with pepper and salt to taste,

and then using a fork, mix well until combined. Set aside to cool.

4. Get a large-sized shallow tray and fill with lukewarm water. One piece at a time, soak the rice paper for a couple of seconds and then put on a clean cutting board. Using a sharp knife, cut the sheet into halves – slice the sheet before it gets completely soft, creating 2 half-circle pieces that are starting to soften.

5. Spoon 1 tablespoon or more of the filling mixture in the corner of 1 sheet. Fold the sheet in alternating directions, making a triangle and then roll the loose ends of the sheet to seal. Repeat the process with the remaining sheets and filling.

6. Put the samosa triangles into the air fryer basket and cook at 200C for 6 minutes.

7. Serve right away.

### 152. Ginger Tahini Noodles With Sesame Crunch Tofu

Servings:3
Cooking Time: 20 Minutes Fry: 392°f
**Ingredients:**
- Sesame Crunch Tofu
- 1 (29-ounce) package bean thread noodles (3 "nests"; see Ingredient Tip)
- 3 tablespoons mellow white miso
- 3 tablespoons tahini (ground sesame paste)
- 3 tablespoons fresh lime juice
- 3 tablespoons grated fresh ginger
- 5 large garlic cloves, minced or pressed
- 1½ cups finely chopped cabbage (red or green, your choice)
- 1½ cups diced cucumber
- ½ cup chopped cilantro
- ⅓ cup finely chopped scallions

**Directions:**
1. Prepare the Sesame Crunch Tofu.
2. While the tofu is cooking, you can get the rest of the dish together. Begin by cooking the noodles according to the directions on the package. (For bean threads, I bring water to a boil, add the nests so they're covered with the water, remove from heat and let sit, covered,

for 5 minutes—or until the noodles are tender.)

3. In a large bowl, add the miso, tahini, and lime juice. Stir well to thoroughly combine, using a wire whisk or fork. Add the ginger and garlic and stir again.

4. Add the cabbage, cucumber, cilantro, and scallions to the bowl. Add the noodles to the bowl, and stir well. Serve topped with the tofu.

### 153. Smooth Mashed Potatoes

Servings: 4
Cooking Time: 25 Minutes
**Ingredients:**
- 4 large potatoes, peeled and cubed
- 1 fresh sprig rosemary
- 2 garlic cloves
- 1 cup vegetable broth
- 1/4 cup almond milk
- 2 tbsp olive oil

**Directions:**
1. Add potatoes, rosemary, garlic, and broth into the inner pot of instant pot duo crisp and stir well.
2. Seal the pot with pressure cooking lid and cook on high for 25 minutes.
3. Once done, release pressure using a quick release. Remove lid.
4. Drain potatoes well and transfer to the large bowl. Remove rosemary sprig.
5. Add oil and almond milk and using potato masher mash the potatoes until smooth.
6. Serve warm and enjoy.

**Vegetables And Sides Recipes**

### 154. Sweet Potato Chips

Servings: 4
Cooking Time: 15 Minutes
**Ingredients:**
- 1 sweet potato, sliced into thin rounds
- 1 bowl water
- 1 tablespoon olive oil
- Salt and pepper to taste
- Cooking spray

**Directions:**
1. Soak sweet potato slices in a bowl of water for 30 minutes.
2. Drain and then dry with paper towels.
3. Toss in oil and season with salt and pepper.
4. Spray air fryer basket with oil.
5. Cook sweet potato at 350 degrees F for 15 minutes, shaking every 5 minutes.

### 155. Herbed Tomatoes With Jalapeno

Servings: 8
Cooking Time: 15 Minutes
**Ingredients:**
- 1 jalapeno pepper, chopped
- 4 garlic cloves, minced
- 2 pounds cherry tomatoes, halved
- Salt and black pepper to the taste
- ¼ cup olive oil
- ½ teaspoon oregano, dried
- ¼ cup basil, chopped

**Directions:**
1. In a bowl, mix tomatoes with garlic, jalapeno, salt, pepper, oregano and the oil, toss to coat, transfer them to your air fryer and cook at 380 degrees F for 15 minutes.
2. Divide fried tomatoes between plates, sprinkle basil on top and serve as a side dish.
3. Enjoy!

### 156. Baby Potatoes Salad

Servings: 4
Cooking Time: 20 Minutes
**Ingredients:**
- 1 and ½ pounds baby potatoes, halved
- 2 garlic cloves, chopped
- 2 red onions, chopped
- 9 ounces cherry tomatoes
- 3 tablespoons olive oil
- 1 and ½ tablespoons balsamic vinegar
- 2 thyme springs, chopped
- Salt and black pepper to the taste

**Directions:**
1. In your food processor, mix garlic with onions, oil, vinegar, thyme, salt and pepper and pulse really well.
2. In a bowl, mix potatoes with tomatoes and balsamic mix, toss, transfer to your air fryer and cook at 380 degrees F for 20 minutes.
3. Divide between plates and serve cold as a side dish.
4. Enjoy!

### 157. Easy Portobello Mushrooms

Servings: 4
Cooking Time: 12 Minutes
**Ingredients:**
- 4 big Portobello mushroom caps
- 1 tablespoon olive oil
- 1 cup spinach, torn
- 1/3 cup vegan breadcrumbs
- ¼ teaspoon rosemary, chopped

**Directions:**
1. Rub mushrooms caps with the oil, place them in your Air Fryer's basket and cook them at 350 ° F for 2 minutes.
2. Meanwhile, in a bowl, mix spinach, rosemary and breadcrumbs and stir well.
3. Stuff mushrooms with this mix, place them in your Air Fryer's basket again and cook at 350 ° F for 10 minutes.
4. Divide them between plates and serve as a side dish.

### 158. Rice With Veggies And Coconut Cream

Servings: 4
Cooking Time: 10 Minutes
**Ingredients:**
- 2 cups rice, cooked
- 1 tablespoon olive oil
- Salt and black pepper to the taste
- 4 garlic cloves, minced
- 2 tablespoons carrot, chopped
- 3 tablespoons small broccoli florets
- 10 tablespoon coconut cream

**Directions:**
1. Preheat your air fryer to 350 degrees F, add oil, garlic, carrots, broccoli, salt and pepper and toss.

2. Add rice and coconut cream, toss, cover and cook for 10 minutes.
3. Divide Rice with Veggies and Coconut Cream between plates and serve as a side dish.
4. Enjoy!

### 159. Yellow Lentils Herbed Mix

Servings: 2
Cooking Time: 15 Minutes
**Ingredients:**
- 1 cup yellow lentils, soaked in water for 1 hour and drained
- 1 hot chili pepper, chopped
- 1-inch ginger piece, grated
- ½ teaspoon turmeric powder
- 1 teaspoon garam masala
- Salt and black pepper to the taste
- 2 teaspoons olive oil
- ½ cup cilantro, chopped
- 1 and ½ cup spinach, chopped
- 4 garlic cloves, minced
- ¾ cup red onion, chopped

**Directions:**
1. In a pan that fits your air fryer, mix lentils with chili pepper, ginger, turmeric, garam masala, salt, pepper, olive oil, cilantro, spinach, onion and garlic, toss, introduce in your air fryer and cook at 400 degrees F for 15 minutes.
2. Divide lentils mix between plates and serve as a side dish.
3. Enjoy!

### 160. Baby Bok Choy

Servings: 4
Cooking Time: 5 minutes
**Ingredients:**
- 1 tsp of garlic powder
- Spray oil
- 4 bunches of baby bok choy

**Directions:**
1. Start by cutting off the bottoms of the four baby bok choy, and proceed to separate their leaves.
2. Rinse well and shake to remove excess water. A bit of dampness is still acceptable. The key is to not have them dripping with water.
3. Move the rinsed bok choy leaves into the air fryer basket and spray with oil

to coat. Sprinkle with some garlic powder and shake to ensure the leaves absorb all the flavor of the garlic.
4. Set the temperature and timer of the air fryer at 350 degrees Fahrenheit for five to six minutes respectively. Shake after two minutes to avoid sticking.

### 161. Corn With Tomatoes Salad

Servings: 4
Cooking Time: 10 Minutes
**Ingredients:**
- 3 cups corn
- A drizzle of olive oil
- Salt and black pepper to the taste
- 1 teaspoon sweet paprika
- 1 tablespoon stevia
- ½ teaspoon garlic powder
- ½ iceberg lettuce head, cut into medium strips
- ½ romaine lettuce head, cut into medium strips
- 1 cup canned black beans, drained
- 3 tablespoons cilantro, chopped
- 4 green onions, chopped
- 12 cherry tomatoes, sliced

**Directions:**
1. Put the corn in a pan that fits your air fryer, drizzle the oil, add salt, pepper, paprika, stevia and garlic powder, introduce in your air fryer and cook at 350 degrees F for 10 minutes.
2. Transfer corn to a salad bowl, add lettuce, black beans, tomatoes, green onions and cilantro, toss, divide between plates and serve as a side salad.
3. Enjoy!

### 162. Spiced Peppers With Jalapenos

Servings: 4
Cooking Time: 16 Minutes
**Ingredients:**
- 4 bell peppers, cut into medium chunks
- ½ cup tomato juice
- 2 tablespoons jarred jalapenos, chopped
- 1 cup tomatoes, chopped
- ¼ cup yellow onion, chopped
- ¼ cup green peppers, chopped
- 2 cups tomato sauce
- Salt and black pepper to the taste
- 2 teaspoons onion powder
- ½ teaspoon red pepper, crushed

- 1 teaspoon chili powder
- ½ teaspoons garlic powder
- 1 teaspoon cumin, ground

**Directions:**
1. In a pan that fits your air fryer, mix tomato juice, jalapenos, tomatoes, onion, green peppers, salt, pepper, onion powder, red pepper, chili powder, garlic powder, oregano and cumin, stir well, introduce in your air fryer and cook at 350 degrees F for 6 minutes
2. Add bell peppers and cook at 320 degrees F for 10 minutes more.
3. Divide peppers mix between plates and serve them as a side dish.
4. Enjoy!

### 163. Mushrooms With Veggies And Avocado

Servings: 2
Cooking Time: 8 Minutes
**Ingredients:**
- 10 ounces mushrooms, halved
- 1 broccoli head, florets separated
- 1 garlic clove, minced
- 1 tablespoon balsamic vinegar
- 1 yellow onion, chopped
- 1 tablespoon olive oil
- Salt and black pepper
- 1 teaspoon basil, dried
- 1 avocado, peeled, pitted and roughly cubed
- A pinch of red pepper flakes

**Directions:**
1. In a bowl, mix mushrooms with broccoli, onion, garlic and avocado.
2. In another bowl, mix vinegar, oil, salt, pepper and basil and whisk well.
3. Pour this over veggies, toss to coat, leave aside for 30 minutes, transfer to your air fryer's basket and cook at 350 degrees F for 8 minutes,
4. Divide between plates and serve with pepper flakes on top as a side dish.
5. Enjoy!

### 164. Cajun Onion With Coconut Cream

Servings: 4
Cooking Time: 15 Minutes
**Ingredients:**
- 2 big white onions, cut into medium chunks
- Salt and black pepper to the taste

- ¼ cup coconut cream
- A drizzle of olive oil
- 1 and ½ teaspoon paprika
- 1 teaspoon garlic powder
- ½ teaspoon Cajun seasoning

**Directions:**
1. In a pan that fits your air fryer, combine onion chunks with salt, pepper, cream, oil, paprika, garlic powder and Cajun seasoning, toss, introduce the pan in your air fryer and cook at 360 degrees F for 15 minutes.
2. Divide the onion mix between plates and serve as a side dish.
3. Enjoy!

### 165. Brussels Sprouts Mix

Servings: 8
Cooking Time: 30 Minutes
**Ingredients:**
- 3 pounds Brussels sprouts, halved
- A drizzle of olive oil
- 4 shallots, chopped
- 4 tablespoons whole wheat flour
- Salt and black pepper to the taste
- 1 cup coconut cream
- 4 tablespoons horseradish
- ¼ teaspoon nutmeg, ground
- 1 tablespoon thyme, chopped

**Directions:**
1. In a bowl, mix sprouts with a drizzle of oil, salt and pepper, toss to coat, put in your air fryer, cook at 400 degrees F for 20 minutes and transfer to a pan that fits your fryer.
2. Add shallots, flour mixed with coconut cream, nutmeg and thyme, toss, put the pan into the fryer and cook at 400 degrees F for 10 minutes more.
3. Divide sprouts mix between plates, top with horseradish and serve as a side dish.
4. Enjoy!

### 166. Baked Tofu Strips

Servings: 4
Cooking Time: 40 Minutes
**Ingredients:**
- 2 tablespoons olive oil
- ½ teaspoon oregano
- ½ teaspoon basil
- ¼ teaspoon cayenne pepper

- ¼ teaspoon paprika
- ¼ teaspoon garlic powder
- ¼ teaspoon onion powder
- Salt and pepper to taste
- 15 oz. tofu, drained

**Directions:**
1. Combine all the ingredients except the tofu.
2. Mix well.
3. Slice tofu into strips and dry with paper towel.
4. Marinate in the mixture for 10 minutes.
5. Cook in the air fryer at 375 degrees F for 15 minutes, shaking halfway through.

### 167. Crispy Vegetables

Servings: 4
Cooking Time: 8 Minutes
**Ingredients:**
- 1 cup rice flour
- 1 tablespoon nutritional yeast flakes
- 2 tablespoons vegan egg powder
- 2/3 cup cold water
- 1 cup breadcrumbs
- Salt and pepper to taste
- 1 cup squash, sliced into strips
- 1 cup zucchini, sliced into strips
- ½ cup green beans
- ½ cup cauliflower, sliced into florets
- Cooking spray

**Directions:**
1. Set up three bowls.
2. One is for the rice flour, another for the egg powder, nutritional yeast and water, another for the breadcrumbs.
3. Dip each of the vegetable slices in the first, second and third bowls.
4. Spray the air fryer basket with oil.
5. Cook at 380 degrees F for 8 minutes or until crispy.

### 168. Cherry Tomatoes Mix

Servings: 4
Cooking Time: 15 Minutes
**Ingredients:**
- 1 tablespoon shallot, chopped
- 1 garlic clove, minced
- ¾ cup cashews, soaked for a couple of hours and drained
- 2 tablespoons nutritional yeast
- ½ cup veggie stock
- Salt and black pepper to the taste

- 2 teaspoons lemon juice
- 1 cup cherry tomatoes, halved
- 5 teaspoons olive oil
- ¼ teaspoon garlic powder

**Directions:**
1. Place tomatoes in a pan that fits your air fryer, drizzle the oil over them, season with salt, black pepper and garlic powder, toss to coat and cook in your air fryer at 350 degrees F for 15 minutes.
2. Meanwhile, in a food processor, mix garlic with shallots, cashews, veggie stock, nutritional yeast, lemon juice, a pinch of sea salt and black pepper to the taste and blend well.
3. Divide tomatoes between plates, drizzle the sauce over them and serve as a side dish.
4. Enjoy!

### 169. Brussels Sprouts With Coconut Cream

Servings: 4
Cooking Time: 10 Minutes
**Ingredients:**
- 1 pound Brussels sprouts, trimmed
- Salt and black pepper to the taste
- 1 tablespoon mustard
- 2 tablespoons coconut cream
- 2 tablespoons dill, chopped

**Directions:**
1. Put Brussels sprouts in your air fryer's basket and cook them at 350 degrees F for 10 minutes.
2. In a bowl, mix cream with mustard, dill, salt and pepper and whisk.
3. Add Brussels sprouts, toss, divide between plates and serve as a side dish.
4. Enjoy!

### 170. Creamy Zucchinis

Servings: 6
Cooking Time: 14 Minutes
**Ingredients:**
- 6 zucchinis, halved and sliced
- Salt and black pepper to the taste
- 1 tablespoon olive oil
- 1 teaspoon oregano, dried
- ½ cup yellow onion, chopped
- 3 garlic cloves, minced
- ¾ cup coconut cream

**Directions:**

1. Heat up a pan that fits your air fryer with the oil over medium-high heat, add onion, stir and cook for 4 minutes.
2. Add garlic, zucchinis, oregano, salt, pepper and cream, toss, introduce in your air fryer and cook at 350 degrees F for 10 minutes.
3. Divide between plates and serve as a side dish.
4. Enjoy!

### 171. Rosemary Potatoes

Servings: 4
Cooking Time: 15 Minutes
**Ingredients:**
- 4 potatoes, cubed
- 1 tablespoon oil
- 1 tablespoon garlic, minced
- 2 teaspoons dried rosemary, minced
- Salt and pepper to taste
- 1 tablespoon lime juice
- ¼ cup parsley, chopped

**Directions:**
1. Toss potato cubes in oil and season with garlic, rosemary, salt and pepper.
2. Put in the air fryer.
3. Cook at 400 degrees F for 15 minutes.
4. Stir in lime juice and top with parsley before serving.

### 172. Crispy Parmesan French Fries

Servings 4
Cooking Time: 10 Minutes
**Ingredients:**
- 390°F FRY
- 4 cups frozen thin French fries
- 2 teaspoons olive oil
- ⅓ cup grated Parmesan cheese
- ½ teaspoon dried thyme
- ½ teaspoon dried basil
- ½ teaspoon salt

**Directions:**
1. If there is any ice on the French fries, remove it. Place the French fries in the air fryer basket and drizzle with the olive oil. Toss gently.
2. Air-fry for about 10 minutes, or until the fries are golden brown and hot, shaking the basket once during cooking time.
3. Immediately put the fries into a serving bowl and sprinkle with the Parmesan,

thyme, basil, and salt. Shake to coat and serve hot.
4. Ingredient tip: Russet potatoes are the best for making French fries because they are low in moisture and bake up tender and crisp. You can use red potatoes or Yukon gold potatoes, but your results won't be quite as crisp.

### 173. Roasted Brussels Sprouts

Servings 4
Cooking Time: 20 Minutes
**Ingredients:**
- 330°F ROAST
- 1 pound fresh Brussels sprouts
- 1 tablespoon olive oil
- ½ teaspoon salt
- ⅛ teaspoon pepper
- ¼ cup grated Parmesan cheese

**Directions:**
1. Trim the bottoms from the Brussels sprouts and pull off any discolored leaves. Toss with the olive oil, salt, and pepper, and place in the air fryer basket.
2. Roast for 20 minutes, shaking the air fryer basket twice during cooking time, until the Brussels sprouts are dark golden brown and crisp.
3. Transfer the Brussels sprouts to a serving dish and toss with the Parmesan cheese. Serve immediately.
4. Did You Know? Brussels sprouts were cultivated in Roman times and introduced into the United States in the 1880s. Most Brussels sprouts in this country are grown in California.

### 174. Creamy Artichokes

Servings: 6
Cooking Time: 6 Minutes
**Ingredients:**
- 14 ounces canned artichoke hearts
- 8 ounces coconut cream
- 10 ounces spinach
- ½ cup veggie stock
- 3 garlic cloves, minced
- ½ cup avocado mayonnaise
- 1 teaspoon onion powder

**Directions:**
1. In a pan that fits your air fryer, mix artichokes with stock, garlic, spinach, cream, onion powder and mayo, toss,

introduce in your air fryer and cook at 350 degrees F for 6 minutes.
2. Divide between plates and serve as a side dish.
3. Enjoy!

### 175. Minty Leeks Medley

Servings: 4
Cooking Time: 12 Minutes
**Ingredients:**
- 6 leeks, roughly chopped
- 1 tablespoon cumin, ground
- 1 tablespoon mint, chopped
- 1 tablespoon parsley, chopped
- 1 teaspoon garlic, minced
- A drizzle of olive oil
- Salt and black pepper to the taste

**Directions:**
1. In a pan that fits your air fryer, combine leeks with cumin, mint, parsley, garlic, salt, pepper and the oil, toss, introduce in your air fryer and cook at 350 degrees F for 12 minutes.
2. Divide Minty Leeks Medley between plates and serve as a side dish.
3. Enjoy!

### 176. Hassel Back Potatoes

Servings: 2
Cooking Time: 40 minutes
**Ingredients:**
- A pinch of black pepper
- 1/4 cup of vegan parmesan cheese (alternatively, use a homemade variety)
- 2 potatoes (russet variety)
- 1/4 tsp of salt
- 2 tbsp of olive oil (extra virgin variety: alternatively, use sub melted non-dairy butter)
- 1/4 cup of mushrooms (Portobello variety: slice thinly)

**Directions:**
1. Start by peeling the potatoes and cut them into thin slices, but not all the way through. The slices should be around 1/8 to 1/4 inch thick.
2. Fill each slot with a thin slice of mushroom.
3. Put the potatoes into the air fryer and brush to coat with half the volume of oil.

4. Set the time and temperature of the air fryer to 20 minutes and 350 degrees Fahrenheit respectively.
5. When the timer elapses, take out the potatoes and sprinkle with pepper and salt. Sprinkle with vegan parmesan cheese as generously as you desire. The nut-free variety of this cheese works best with this recipe.

### 177. Kale Chips

Servings: 2
Cooking Time: 10 Minutes
**Ingredients:**
- Cooking spray
- 6 cups kale leaves, torn
- 1 tablespoon olive oil
- Salt to taste
- 1 ½ teaspoons low-sodium soy sauce
- ¼ teaspoon ground cumin
- ½ teaspoon white sesame seeds

**Directions:**
1. Spray air fryer basket with oil.
2. Toss kale in oil, salt and soy sauce.
3. Cook at 375 degrees F for 10 minutes or until crispy. Shake every 3 minutes.
4. Sprinkle with cumin and sesame seeds before serving.

### 178. Collard Greens And Tomatoes

Servings: 4
Cooking Time: 10 Minutes
**Ingredients:**
- 1 pound collard greens
- ¼ cup cherry tomatoes, halved
- 1 tablespoon apple cider vinegar
- 2 tablespoons veggie stock
- Salt and black pepper to the taste

**Directions:**
1. In a pan that fits your Air Fryer, combine tomatoes, collard greens, vinegar, stock, salt and pepper, stir, introduce in your Air Fryer and cook at 320 ° F for 10 minutes.
2. Divide between plates and serve as a side dish.

### 179. Spiced Cauliflower Rice

Servings: 4
Cooking Time: 20 Minutes
**Ingredients:**
- 4 tablespoons coconut aminos

- ½ block firm tofu, cubed
- 1 cup carrot, chopped
- ½ cup yellow onion, chopped
- 1 teaspoon turmeric powder
- 3 cups cauliflower, riced
- 1 and ½ teaspoons sesame oil
- 1 tablespoon rice vinegar
- ½ cup broccoli florets, chopped
- 1 tablespoon ginger, minced
- 2 garlic cloves, minced
- ½ cup peas

**Directions:**
1. In a bowl, mix tofu with 2 tablespoons coconut aminos, ½ cup onion, turmeric and carrot, toss to coat, transfer into your air fryer and cook at 370 degrees F for 10 minutes, shaking halfway.
2. In a bowl, mix cauliflower rice with the rest of the coconut aminos, sesame oil, garlic, vinegar, ginger, broccoli and peas, stir, add to the tofu mix from the fryer, toss and cook everything at 370 degrees F for 10 minutes.
3. Divide between plates and serve as a side dish.
4. Enjoy!

### 180. Tomatoes With Basil And Garlic

Servings: 2
Cooking Time: 14 Minutes
**Ingredients:**
- 1 bunch basil, chopped
- 3 garlic clove, minced
- A drizzle of olive oil
- Salt and black pepper to the taste
- 2 cups cherry tomatoes, halved

**Directions:**
1. In a pan that fits your air fryer, combine tomatoes with garlic, salt, pepper, basil and oil, toss, introduce in your air fryer and cook at 320 degrees F for 12 minutes.
2. Divide between plates and serve as a side dish.
3. Enjoy!

### 181. Creamy Zucchini And Sweet Potatoes

Servings: 8
Cooking Time: 16 Minutes
**Ingredients:**
- 1 cup veggie stock

- 2 tablespoons olive oil
- 2 sweet potatoes, peeled and cut into medium wedges
- 8 zucchinis, cut into medium wedges
- 2 yellow onions, chopped
- 1 cup coconut milk
- Salt and black pepper to the taste
- 1 tablespoon coconut aminos
- ¼ teaspoon thyme, dried
- ¼ teaspoon rosemary, dried
- 4 tablespoons dill, chopped
- ½ teaspoon basil, chopped

**Directions:**
1. Heat up a pan that fits your air fryer with the oil over medium heat, add onion, stir and cook for 2 minutes.
2. Add zucchinis, thyme, rosemary, basil, potato, salt, pepper, stock, milk, aminos and dill, stir, introduce in your air fryer, cook at 360 degrees F for 14 minutes, divide between plates and serve as a side dish.
3. Enjoy!

### 182. Scalloped Potatoes

Servings 4
Cooking Time: 20 Minutes
**Ingredients:**
- 380°F BAKE
- 2 cups pre-sliced refrigerated potatoes
- 3 cloves garlic, minced
- Pinch salt
- Freshly ground black pepper
- ¾ cup heavy cream

**Directions:**
1. Layer the potatoes, garlic, salt, and pepper in a 6-by-6-by-2-inch baking pan. Slowly pour the cream over all.
2. Bake for 15 minutes, until the potatoes are golden brown on top and tender. Check their state and, if needed, bake for 5 minutes until browned.
3. Ingredient tip: You can top these potatoes with cheese after about 10 minutes of baking time. Add ⅔ cup of shredded Swiss, Havarti, or Gouda, and bake until the cheese is bubbling and starts to brown.

### 183. Easy Peppers Side Dish

Servings: 12
Cooking Time: 25 Minutes

**Ingredients:**
- 12 colored bell peppers, seedless and sliced
- 1 tablespoon olive oil
- 1 yellow onion, sliced
- ½ teaspoon smoked paprika
- Salt and black pepper to the taste

**Directions:**
1. Put the oil in a pan that fits your Air Fryer, add bell peppers, paprika and onion, toss, introduce the pan in your Air Fryer and cook at 320 ° F for 25 minutes.
2. Season with salt and pepper to the taste, divide between plates and serve as a side dish.

### 184. Red Potatoes And Green Beans

Servings: 4
Cooking Time: 15 Minutes
**Ingredients:**
- 1 pound red potatoes, cut into wedges
- 1 pound green beans
- 2 garlic cloves, minced
- 2 tablespoons olive oil
- Salt and black pepper to the taste
- ½ teaspoon oregano, dried

**Directions:**
1. In a pan that fits your Air Fryer, combine potatoes with green beans, garlic, oil, salt, pepper and oregano, toss, introduce in your Air Fryer and cook at 380 ° F for 15 minutes.
2. Divide between plates and serve as a side dish.

### 185. Plums With Almonds And Stevia

Servings: 4
Cooking Time: 12 Minutes
**Ingredients:**
- 3 tablespoons stevia
- 3 ounces almonds, peeled and chopped
- 12 ounces plumps, pitted
- 2 tablespoons veggie stock
- 2 yellow onions, chopped
- 2 garlic cloves, minced
- Salt and black pepper to the tastes
- 1 teaspoon cumin powder
- 1 teaspoon turmeric powder
- 1 teaspoon ginger powder
- 1 teaspoon cinnamon powder

- 3 tablespoons olive oil

**Directions:**
1. In a pan that fits your air fryer, combine almonds with plums, stevia, stock, onions, garlic, salt, pepper, cumin, turmeric, ginger, cinnamon and oil, toss, introduce in your air fryer and cook at 350 degrees F for 12 minutes.
2. Divide plums mix between plates and serve as a side dish
3. Enjoy!

### 186. Long Beans Mix

Servings: 3
Cooking Time: 10 Minutes
**Ingredients:**
- ½ teaspoon coconut aminos
- 1 tablespoon olive oil
- A pinch of salt and black pepper
- 4 garlic cloves, minced
- 4 long beans, trimmed and sliced

**Directions:**
1. In a pan that fits your Air Fryer, combine long beans with oil, aminos, salt, pepper and garlic, toss, introduce in your Air Fryer and cook at 350° F for 10 minutes.
2. Divide between plates and serve as a side dish.

### 187. Creamy Corn Casserole

Servings 4
Cooking Time: 15 Minutes
**Ingredients:**
- 320°F BAKE
- Nonstick baking spray with flour
- 2 cups frozen yellow corn
- 3 tablespoons flour
- 1 egg, beaten
- ¼ cup milk
- ½ cup light cream
- ½ cup grated Swiss or Havarti cheese
- Pinch salt
- Freshly ground black pepper
- 2 tablespoons butter, cut in cubes

**Directions:**
1. Spray a 6-by-6-by-2-inch baking pan with nonstick spray.
2. In a medium bowl, combine the corn, flour, egg, milk, and light cream, and mix until combined. Stir in the cheese, salt, and pepper.

3. Pour this mixture into the prepared baking pan. Dot with the butter.
4. Bake for 15 minutes.
5. Substitution tip: You can substitute one 15-ounce can of corn, drained, for the frozen corn. Or cut the kernels off 2 to 3 ears of corn to use in this recipe.

### 188. Savory Roasted Sweet Potatoes

Servings 4
Cooking Time: 25 Minutes
**Ingredients:**
- 330°F ROAST
- 2 sweet potatoes, peeled and cut into 1-inch cubes
- 1 tablespoon olive oil
- Pinch salt
- Freshly ground black pepper
- ½ teaspoon dried thyme
- ½ teaspoon dried marjoram
- ¼ cup grated Parmesan cheese

**Directions:**
1. Put the sweet potato cubes in the air fryer basket and drizzle with the olive oil. Toss gently. Sprinkle with the salt, pepper, thyme, and marjoram, and toss again.
2. Roast for 20 minutes, shaking the air fryer basket once during cooking time.
3. Remove the basket from the air fryer and shake the potatoes again. Sprinkle evenly with the Parmesan cheese and return to the air fryer.
4. Roast for 5 minutes or until the potatoes are tender.
5. Did You Know? Sweet potatoes and yams are two different types of root vegetable. A true yam is a starchy white root vegetable used in Caribbean cooking. Sweet potatoes are high in vitamin A and are usually bright orange in color.

### 189. Crispy Air Fryer Sweet Potato Tots

Servings: 25
Cooking Time: 12 minutes
**Ingredients:**
- Spray oil
- 1/2 tsp of coriander
- 2 cups of puree (sweet potato variety)
- 1/2 tsp of cumin

- 1/2 cup of regular bread crumbs or panko bread crumbs
- 1/2 tsp of salt

**Directions:**
1. Start by preheating the air fryer to a temperature of 390 degrees Fahrenheit.
2. Get a large-sized bowl and pour in all the ingredients. Mix to combine well.
3. Use a cookie scoop to form a tablespoon of tots and lay it out on one to two plates.
4. Use the spray oil to coat the tots and move them carefully to coat their bottoms with a layer of oil, too.
5. Take care to arrange the tots into the air fryer basket in such a way that there is enough space between them. You might have to prepare them in two to three batches.
6. Proceed to cook the tots for six to seven minutes, taking care to turn them over gently. When the tots feel mushy and soft when you flip them over, let them cook for another few minutes.
7. Set the timer to cook for another five to seven minutes, or until both sides of the tots become crispy but not burned.
8. When done, serve immediately with chipotle mayonnaise, ketchup, or guacamole as dip.

### 190. Creamy Brussels Sprouts

Servings: 4
Cooking Time: 10 Minutes
**Ingredients:**
- 1 pound Brussels sprouts, trimmed
- Salt and black pepper to the taste
- 1 tablespoon mustard
- 2 tablespoons coconut cream
- 2 tablespoons dill, chopped

**Directions:**
1. Put Brussels sprouts in your Air Fryer's basket and cook them at 350 ° F for 10 minutes.
2. In a bowl, mix cream with mustard, dill, salt and pepper and whisk.
3. Add Brussels sprouts, toss, divide between plates and serve as a side dish.

### 191. Chili Fennel

Servings: 4
Cooking Time: 8 Minutes
**Ingredients:**

- 2 fennel bulbs, cut into quarters
- 3 tablespoons olive oil
- Salt and black pepper to the taste
- 1 garlic clove, minced
- 1 red chili pepper, chopped
- ¾ cup veggie stock
- Juice of ½ lemon

**Directions:**
1. Heat up a pan that fits your Air Fryer with the oil over medium-high heat, add garlic and chili pepper, stir and cook for 2 minutes.
2. Add fennel, salt, pepper, stock and lemon juice, toss to coat, introduce in your Air Fryer and cook at 350 ° F for 6 minutes.
3. Divide between plates and serve as a side dish.

### 192. Fennel With Red Chili

Servings: 4
Cooking Time: 8 Minutes
**Ingredients:**
- 2 fennel bulbs, cut into quarters
- 3 tablespoons olive oil
- Salt and black pepper to the taste
- 1 garlic clove, minced
- 1 red chili pepper, chopped
- ¾ cup veggie stock
- Juice of ½ lemon

**Directions:**
1. Heat up a pan that fits your air fryer with the oil over medium-high heat, add garlic and chili pepper, stir and cook for 2 minutes.
2. Add fennel, salt, pepper, stock and lemon juice, toss to coat, introduce in your air fryer and cook at 350 degrees F for 6 minutes.
3. Divide between plates and serve as a side dish.
4. Enjoy!

### 193. Potatoes With Green Beans

Servings: 4
Cooking Time: 15 Minutes
**Ingredients:**
- 1 pound red potatoes, cut into wedges
- 1 pound green beans
- 2 garlic cloves, minced
- 2 tablespoons olive oil
- Salt and black pepper to the taste

- ½ teaspoon oregano, dried

**Directions:**
1. In a pan that fits your air fryer, combine potatoes with green beans, garlic, oil, salt, pepper and oregano, toss, introduce in your air fryer and cook at 380 degrees F for 15 minutes.
2. Divide between plates and serve as a side dish.
3. Enjoy!

### 194. Roasted Spicy Carrots

Servings: 4
Cooking Time: 15 Minutes
**Ingredients:**
- ½ lb. carrots, sliced
- ½ tablespoon olive oil
- Salt to taste
- 1/8 teaspoon garlic powder
- ¼ teaspoon chili powder
- 1 teaspoon ground cumin
- Sesame seeds
- Fresh cilantro

**Directions:**
1. Preheat your air fryer at 390 degrees F for 5 minutes.
2. Cook the carrots at 390 degrees F for 10 minutes.
3. Transfer to a bowl.
4. Mix the oil, salt, garlic powder, chili powder and ground cumin.
5. Coat the carrots with the oil mixture.
6. Put the carrots back to the air fryer and cook for another 5 minutes.
7. Garnish with sesame seeds and cilantro.

### 195. Baked Potatoes With Broccoli & Cheese

Servings: 8
Cooking Time: 30 Minutes
**Ingredients:**
- 4 potatoes
- 1 cup almond milk, divided
- 2 tablespoons all-purpose flour
- ½ cup vegan cheese, divided
- 1 cup broccoli, florets, chopped
- Salt to taste
- Chopped onion chives

**Directions:**
1. Poke all sides of potatoes with a fork.
2. Microwave on high level for 5 minutes.
3. Flip and microwave for another 5 minutes.

4. In a saucepan over medium heat, heat ¾ cup of milk for 2 minutes, stirring frequently.
5. Add the remaining milk in a bowl and stir in the flour.
6. Add this mixture to the pan and bring to a boil.
7. Reduce heat
8. Reserve 2 tablespoons vegan cheese.
9. Add the rest of the cheese to the pan and stir until smooth.
10. Add the broccoli, salt and cayenne.
11. Cook for 1 minute and remove from heat.
12. Slice the potatoes and arrange on a single layer inside the air fryer.
13. Top with the broccoli mixture.
14. Add another layer of potatoes and broccoli mixture.
15. Sprinkle reserved cheese on top.
16. Cook at 350 degrees F for 5 minutes.
17. Garnish with chopped chives.

### 196. Steamed Green Veggie Trio

Servings 4
Cooking Time: 9 Minutes
**Ingredients:**
- 330°F STEAM
- FAST, VEGAN, GLUTEN-FREE
- 2 cups broccoli florets
- 1 cup green beans
- 1 tablespoon olive oil
- 1 tablespoon lemon juice
- 1 cup frozen baby peas
- 2 tablespoons honey mustard
- Pinch salt
- Freshly ground black pepper

**Directions:**
1. Put the broccoli and green beans in the basket of the air fryer. Put 2 tablespoons water in the air fryer pan. Sprinkle the vegetables with the olive oil and lemon juice, and toss.
2. Steam for 6 minutes, then remove the basket from the air fryer and add the peas.
3. Steam for 3 minutes or until the vegetables are hot and tender.
4. Transfer the vegetables to a serving dish and drizzle with the honey mustard and sprinkle with salt and pepper. Toss and serve.

5. Ingredient tip: To prepare broccoli, cut the florets off the stem. You can freeze the stem to use in stir-fries later. To prepare green beans, cut off both ends and rinse well.

### 197. Beet And Garlic Salad

Servings: 4
Cooking Time: 14 Minutes
**Ingredients:**
- 4 beets, trimmed
- 2 tablespoons balsamic vinegar
- A bunch of parsley, chopped
- Salt and black pepper to the taste
- 1 tablespoon extra virgin olive oil
- 1 garlic clove, chopped
- 2 tablespoons capers

**Directions:**
1. Put beets in your air fryer's basket and cook them at 360 degrees F for 14 minutes.
2. In a bowl, mix parsley with garlic, salt, pepper, olive oil and capers and stir very well.
3. Leave beets to cool down, peel them, slice, put them in a bowl, add vinegar and the parsley mix, toss, divide between plates and serve as a side dish.
4. Enjoy!

### 198. Baby Carrots With Stevia

Servings: 4
Cooking Time: 12 Minutes
**Ingredients:**
- 3 cups baby carrots
- Salt and black pepper to the taste
- 1 tablespoon stevia
- 1 tablespoon olive oil

**Directions:**
1. In a bowl, mix carrots with salt, pepper, oil and stevia, toss to coat, transfer carrots to your air fryer and cook at 400 degrees F for 12 minutes.
2. Divide between plates and serve them as a side dish.
3. Enjoy!

### 199. Root Vegetables With Vegan Aioli

Servings: 4
Cooking Time: 30 Minutes
**Ingredients:**
- To prepare the garlic aioli:

- Salt
- Black pepper (ground)
- 1/2 cup of vegan mayo
- 1/2 tsp of fresh lemon juice
- 1 clove of garlic (minced)
- To prepare the root vegetables:
- 1/2 tsp of lemon zest (grated)
- 4 the of olive oil (extra virgin variety)
- 1/2 lbs of baby red potatoes (cut into four to six pieces lengthwise)
- 3 cloves of garlic (minced finely)
- 1/2 red onion, (cut into half-inch slices lengthwise)
- 1 tbsp of fresh rosemary (minced)
- 1/2 lbs of baby carrots (cut lengthwise)
- 1 tsp of kosher salt
- 1 lbs of parsnips (peel and cut lengthwise into uniform sizes)
- 1/2 tsp of black pepper (ground)

**Directions:**
1. Start by mixing the pepper, salt, lemon juice, garlic, and mayonnaise into a small-sized bowl to prepare the garlic aioli. Store in the refrigerator until completing the recipe.
2. Proceed to preheat the air fryer to a temperature of 400 degrees Fahrenheit.
3. Get another small-sized bowl and begin to mix the rosemary, salt, olive oil, pepper, and garlic. Allow to sit for the flavors to mix. Introduce the rosemary and olive oil mix into the bowl, stirring until the vegetables are well coated. Arrange a portion of veggies into a single file in the air fryer basket before proceeding to include a rack, as well as a second layer of veggies.
4. Set the timer for 15 minutes and air fry the veggies.
5. To prepare the garlic aioli, get a small-sized bowl and pour in the lemon juice. Add the mayonnaise and garlic and sprinkle with pepper and salt. Mix thoroughly and store in the refrigerator until you complete the recipe.
6. Begin preheating the air fryer to 400 degrees F (200 degrees C). This feature is only available if your air fryer model allows preheating. Otherwise, heat as normal.
7. Get a small-sized bowl and pour in the olive oil. Add some garlic and rosemary and sprinkle with pepper and salt. Mix thoroughly and allow to sit for the flavors to combine.
8. Get a large-sized bowl and pour in onion, carrots, parsnips and potatoes. Mix well. Pour in the olive oil and rosemary mix and begin stirring until the vegetables are coated evenly. Arrange the vegetables into a single layer in the air fryer basket. Include another rack to cook another layer of vegetables.
9. When the timer elapses, collect the vegetables into plates and store in a warm place or keep cooking for five-minute intervals, until the vegetables become brown or done as you prefer.
10. Arrange the remaining veggies into the bottom of the basket of the air fryer and run the timer for 15 minutes. Check for level of doneness as necessary. Make use of the rack again to prepare any further remainder of vegetables that can be arranged in single layers. When every vegetable has been successfully cooked, serve with the garlic aioli and lemon zest as garnish.

## 200. Vegan Hush Puppies

Servings: 4
Cooking Time: 10 minutes
**Ingredients:**
- Spray oil (optional)
- 1/4 cup of onion (minced)
- 1/4 cup of soy milk
- 1 cup of cornmeal (ground finely if possible)
- 1/2 tsp of salt
- 1/4 cup of aquafaba
- 1 tbsp of olive oil (use more aquafaba alternatively)
- 1½ tsp of baking powder
- 1 tbsp of vegan sugar or any other vegan sweetener of your choosing
- 1/2 tsp of salt
- 1 tsp of apple cider vinegar (make use of a different Milt to leave out vinegar)

**Directions:**
1. Get a medium-sized mixing bowl and pour in the baking powder and

cornmeal. Sprinkle with salt and mix well to combine.
2. Pour in the olive oil, aquafaba, non-dairy milk, sugar, and onion, mixing them in.
3. Scoop 1 tablespoon of batter and proceed to mold it into a ball. Alternatively, you can try using a 1 tablespoon scoop rather than your hands. Place all of the batter into the air fryer basket.
4. When the air fryer basket gets full, spray the rolled-up batter with oil if preferred, otherwise don't. Set the time and temperature to 10 minutes and 390 degrees Fahrenheit respectively. To prevent sticking, consider using parchment paper or shake the basket after a five-minute interval. Repeat the process until more hush puppies are baked.

### 201. Paprika Broccoli

Servings: 4
Cooking Time: 20 Minutes
**Ingredients:**
- 1 broccoli head, florets separated
- Juice of ½ lemon
- 1 tablespoon olive oil
- 2 teaspoons paprika
- Salt and black pepper to the taste
- 3 garlic cloves, minced
- 1 tablespoon sesame seeds
**Directions:**
1. In a bowl, mix broccoli with lemon juice, oil, paprika, salt, pepper and garlic and toss to coat.
2. Transfer to your Air Fryer's basket, cook at 360 ° F for 15 minutes, sprinkle sesame seeds, cook for 5 minutes more, divide between plates and serve as a side dish.

### 202. Tomatoes And Basil Mix

Servings: 2
Cooking Time: 14 Minutes
**Ingredients:**
- 1 bunch basil, chopped
- 3 garlic clove, minced
- A drizzle of olive oil
- Salt and black pepper to the taste
- 2 cups cherry tomatoes, halved

**Directions:**
1. In a pan that fits your Air Fryer, combine tomatoes with garlic, salt, pepper, basil and oil, toss, introduce in your Air Fryer and cook at 320 ° F for 12 minutes.
2. Divide between plates and serve as a side dish.

### 203. White Mushrooms Mix

Servings: 2
Cooking Time: 15 Minutes
**Ingredients:**
- Salt and black pepper to the taste
- 7 ounces snow peas
- 8 ounces white mushrooms, halved
- 1 yellow onion, cut into rings
- 2 tablespoons coconut aminos
- 1 teaspoon olive oil
**Directions:**
1. In a bowl, snow peas with mushrooms, onion, aminos, oil, salt and pepper, toss well, transfer to a pan that fits your Air Fryer, introduce in the fryer and cook at 350 °F for 15 minutes.
2. Divide between plates and serve as a side dish

### 204. Summer Squash Mix

Servings: 4
Cooking Time: 10 Minutes
**Ingredients:**
- 3 ounces coconut cream
- ½ teaspoon oregano, dried
- Salt and black pepper
- 1 big yellow summer squash, peeled and cubed
- 1/3 cup carrot, cubed
- 2 tablespoons olive oil
**Directions:**
1. In a pan that fits your Air Fryer, combine squash with carrot, oil, oregano, salt, pepper and coconut cream, toss, transfer to your Air Fryer and cook at 400 ° F for 10 minutes.
2. Divide between plates and serve as a side dish.

## Desserts Recipes

### 205. Tangerine Cake

Servings: 8
Cooking Time: 20 Minutes
**Ingredients:**
- ¾ cup coconut sugar
- 2 cups whole wheat flour
- ¼ cup olive oil
- ½ cup almond milk
- 1 teaspoon cider vinegar
- ½ teaspoon vanilla extract
- Juice and zest of 2 lemons
- Juice and zest of 1 tangerine

**Directions:**
1. In a bowl, mix flour with sugar and stir.
2. In another bowl, mix oil with milk, vinegar, vanilla extract, lemon juice and zest, tangerine zest and flour, whisk very well, pour this into a cake pan that fits your air fryer, introduce in the fryer and cook at 360 degrees F for 20 minutes.
3. Serve right away.
4. Enjoy!

### 206. Peach Cobbler

Servings: 4
Cooking Time: 30 Minutes
**Ingredients:**
- 4 cups peaches, peeled and sliced
- ¼ cup coconut sugar
- ½ teaspoon cinnamon powder
- 1 and ½ cups vegan crackers, crushed
- ¼ cup stevia
- ¼ teaspoon nutmeg, ground
- ½ cup almond milk
- 1 teaspoon vanilla extract
- Cooking spray

**Directions:**
1. In a bowl, mix peaches with coconut sugar and cinnamon and stir.
2. In a separate bowl, mix crackers with stevia, nutmeg, almond milk and vanilla extract and stir.
3. Spray a pie pan that fits your air fryer with cooking spray and spread peaches on the bottom.
4. Add crackers mix, spread, introduce into the fryer and cook at 350 degrees F for 30 minutes

5. Divide the cobbler between plates and serve.
6. Enjoy!

### 207. Sweet Apple Cupcakes

Servings: 4
Cooking Time: 20 Minutes
**Ingredients:**
- 4 tablespoons vegetable oil
- 3 tablespoons flax meal combined with 3 tablespoons water
- ½ cup pure applesauce
- 2 teaspoons cinnamon powder
- 1 teaspoon vanilla extract
- 1 apple, cored and chopped
- 4 teaspoons maple syrup
- ¾ cup whole wheat flour
- ½ teaspoon baking powder

**Directions:**
1. Heat up a pan with the oil over medium heat, add applesauce, vanilla, flax meal and maple syrup, stir, take off heat and cool down.
2. Add flour, cinnamon, baking powder and apples, whisk, pour into a cupcake pan, introduce in your air fryer at 350 degrees F and bake for 20 minutes.
3. Transfer cupcakes to a platter and serve them warm.
4. Enjoy!

### 208. Two-sided Cake

Servings: 6
Cooking Time: 60 Minutes
**Ingredients:**
- 100 g / 0.22 lbs rice flour
- 100 g / 0.22 lbs oatmeal flour
- 100 g / 0.4 cup soy milk
- 1 teaspoon vanilla sugar
- 1 teaspoon stevia extract
- 2 teaspoon cocoa
- 10 g / 0.35 oz crushed nuts
- 1 teaspoon olive oil

**Directions:**
1. For this dessert, you should make 2 separate mixtures. Take the big bowl and combine rice flour and 50 g soy milk in it. Stir it carefully. Add vanilla sugar and cocoa. Stir it carefully and knead dough. Then cover the mass with the towel and leave it. Meanwhile, take another bowl and put oatmeal flour

and another 50 g of soy milk in it. Mix it with the hand of the hand mixer. Add stevia extract and crushed nuts. Knead the dough and put it in the freezer for 10 minutes. Meanwhile, preheat the air fryer to 190 C / 380 F. Take the tray and spray it with olive oil. Roll dough and put a flat piece of dough to the tray. Then remove the other piece of dough from the freezer and grate it on the dough layer. Transfer the cake to the air fryer and cook it for 25 minutes more. Then remove the cake from the air fryer and cut it into pieces. Serve it warm but not hot. Enjoy!

### 209. Semolina Cake

Servings: 6
Cooking Time: 30 Minutes
**Ingredients:**
- 1 cup fine farina, milled fine
- 2 cups hot water
- 1 cup dried fruit
- 1 cup sugar
- 1 cup almond milk
- ¼ cup soy yogurt
- ¼ cup coconut oil
- 1 tsp. ground cardamom
- ½ tsp. baking soda
- 1 tsp. baking powder

**Directions:**
1. Soak the dried fruit in hot water and set aside.
2. Grease an 8-inch heat-safe baking pan and keep aside.
3. In a large mixing bowl whisk together the milk, farina, oil, sugar, soy yogurt and cardamom.
4. Set this mixture aside for 20 minutes to allow the farina to soften and absorb the liquid.
5. Drain the dried fruit well, and mix into the batter.
6. Add the baking soda and baking powder and mix well.
7. Pour the cake batter into the prepared cake pan and set the pan into the air fryer basket.
8. Set the air fryer to 330 degrees Fahrenheit for 25 minutes.

9. At the end of the bake time, insert a cake tester to check for doneness. It should come out clean.
10. Remove the pan, let rest for 10 minutes and then unmold the cake.
11. Serve and enjoy!

### 210. Cocoa And Coconut Bars

Servings: 12
Cooking Time: 14 Minutes
**Ingredients:**
- 6 ounces coconut oil, melted
- 3 tablespoons flax meal combined with 3 tablespoons water
- 3 ounces cocoa powder
- 2 teaspoons vanilla
- ½ teaspoon baking powder
- 4 ounces coconut cream
- 5 tablespoons coconut sugar

**Directions:**
1. In a blender, mix flax meal with oil, cocoa powder, baking powder, vanilla, cream and sugar and pulse.
2. Pour this into a lined baking dish that fits your air fryer, introduce in the fryer at 320 degrees F, bake for 14 minutes, slice into rectangles and serve.
3. Enjoy!

### 211. Carrot Mug Cakes

Servings: 1
Cooking Time: 15 Minutes
**Ingredients:**
- ¼ cups whole-wheat, gluten-free pastry flour,
- 1 tbsp. brown sugar or coconut sugar
- ¼ teaspoon ground cinnamon
- ¼ teaspoon baking powder
- 2 tbsp. almond milk plus 2 tsp. more
- 1 tbsp. raisins or chopped dates
- 2 tbsp. grated carrot
- 2 tbsp. chopped walnuts
- 1/8 teaspoon ground dried ginger
- A pinch ground allspice
- A pinch of salt
- 2 tsp. flavorless oil

**Directions:**
1. Lightly oil an oven-safe ceramic mug.
2. Add the flour, baking powder, sugar, ginger, allspice, cinnamon and salt then mix well with a fork.

3. Next add the carrot, milk, walnuts, raisins and oil and then mix again.
4. Bake in an air fryer at 350 degrees Fahrenheit for 15 minutes.
5. Check with a cake tester to make sure the middle is cooked.
6. If not, cook for 5 additional minutes.
7. Serve warm!

### 212. Raspberry Lemon Streusel Cake

Servings:6
Cooking Time: 45 Minutes Bake: 311°f
**Ingredients:**
- For the streusel topping
- 2 tablespoons organic sugar
- 2 tablespoons neutral-flavored oil (sunflower, safflower, or refined coconut)
- ¼ cup plus 2 tablespoons whole-wheat pastry flour (or gluten-free all-purpose flour)
- For the cake
- 1 cup whole-wheat pastry flour
- ½ cup organic sugar
- 1 teaspoon baking powder
- 1 tablespoon lemon zest
- ¼ teaspoon sea salt
- ¾ cup plus 2 tablespoons unsweetened nondairy milk (plain or vanilla)
- 2 tablespoons neutral-flavored oil (sunflower, safflower, or refined coconut)
- 1 teaspoon vanilla
- 1 cup fresh raspberries
- Cooking oil spray (sunflower, safflower, or refined coconut)
- For the icing
- ½ cup powdered sugar
- 1 tablespoon fresh lemon juice
- ½ teaspoon lemon zest
- ½ teaspoon vanilla
- ⅛ teaspoon sea salt

**Directions:**
1. In a medium bowl, place the flour, sugar, baking powder, zest, and salt. Stir very well, preferably with a wire whisk. Add the milk, oil, and vanilla. Stir with a rubber spatula or spoon, just until thoroughly combined. Gently stir in the raspberries.

2. Preheat the air fryer for 3 minutes. Spray or coat the insides of a 6-inch round, 2-inch deep baking pan with oil and pour the batter into the pan.
3. Remove the streusel from the fridge and crumble it over the top of the cake batter. Carefully place the cake in the air fryer and bake for 45 minutes, or until a knife inserted in the center comes out clean (the top should be golden-brown).
4. To make the icing
5. In a small bowl, stir together the powdered sugar, lemon juice and zest, vanilla, and salt. Once the cake has cooled for about 5 minutes, slice into 4 pieces and drizzle each with icing. Serve warm if possible. If you have leftovers, they will keep in an airtight container in the fridge for several days.

### 213. Cinnamon Apples And Mandarin Sauce

Servings: 4
Cooking Time: 20 Minutes
**Ingredients:**
- 4 apples, cored, peeled and cored
- 2 cups mandarin juice
- ¼ cup maple syrup
- 2 teaspoons cinnamon powder
- 1 tablespoon ginger, grated

**Directions:**
1. In a pan that fits your air fryer, mix apples with mandarin juice, maple syrup, cinnamon and ginger, introduce in the fryer and cook at 365 degrees F for 20 minutes
2. Divide apples mix between plates and serve warm.
3. Enjoy!

### 214. Stuffed Apples

Servings:  5
Cooking Time: 25 Minutes
**Ingredients:**
- 5 apples, tops cut off and cored
- 5 figs
- 1/3 cup coconut sugar
- ¼ cup pecans, chopped
- 2 teaspoons lemon zest, grated
- ½ teaspoon cinnamon powder
- 1 tablespoon lemon juice
- 1tablespoon coconut oil

**Directions:**

1. In a bowl mix figs, coconut sugar, pecans, lemon zest, cinnamon, lemon juice and coconut oil and stir.
2. Stuff the apples with this mix, introduce them in your air fryer and cook at 365 degrees F for 25 minutes.
3. Enjoy!

### 215. De-light-full Caramelized Apples

Servings:2
Cooking Time: 20 Minutes Bake: 392°f
**Ingredients:**

- 2 apples, any sweet variety
- 2 tablespoons water
- 1½ teaspoons coconut sugar
- ¼ teaspoon cinnamon
- Pinch nutmeg
- Dash sea salt
- Cooking oil spray (sunflower, safflower, or refined coconut)

**Directions:**

1. Cut each apple in half (no need to peel) and then remove the core and seeds, doing your best to keep the apple halves intact—because ideally, you want apple halves, not quarters.
2. Place the apples upright in a 6-inch round, 2-inch deep baking pan. Add about 2 tablespoons water to the bottom of the dish to keep the apples from drying out (the apples will sit in the water).
3. Sprinkle the tops of the apples evenly with the sugar, cinnamon, and nutmeg. Give each half a very light sprinkle of sea salt.
4. In short spurts, spray the tops with oil (if you spray too hard, it will make the toppings fly off in a tragic whirlwind). Once moistened, spray the tops again with oil. (This will keep them from drying out.)
5. Bake for 20 minutes, or until the apples are very soft and nicely browned on top. Enjoy immediately, plain or topped with granola and/or ice cream.

### 216. Black Currant Pudding-cake

Servings: 6
Cooking Time: 50 Minutes
**Ingredients:**

- 100 g / 0.22 lbs rice flour

- 2 tablespoon soy milk
- 1 teaspoon baking soda
- 100 g / 0.4 cup water
- 3 tablespoon almond milk
- 100 g / 0.22 lbs black currant
- 1 teaspoon stevia extract
- 1 teaspoon oatmeal flour
- 40 g / 1.4 oz apple puree

**Directions:**

1. Take the bowl and combine rice flour and soy milk together. Add baking soda and almond milk. Stir it and add oatmeal flour and stevia extract. Then add water. Mix the mass with the help of the hand mixer till it smooth. Then knead dough. Take the black currant and transfer it to the blender. Blend it for 3 minutes and add apple puree. Blend it for 3 minutes more. Then preheat the air fryer to 200 C / 390 F, put the flat tray in it and pour the currant mass. Close the lid and reduce the temperature to 150 C / 300 F and cook it for 30 minutes. Then remove the dish from the air fryer and chill it. Cut it into pieces and serve it immediately. Enjoy!

### 217. Cranberry Pudding

Servings:   4
Cooking Time: 30 Minutes
**Ingredients:**

- 4 ounces dried cranberries, chopped
- A drizzle of olive oil
- 4 ounces dried apricots, chopped
- 1 cup white flour
- 3 teaspoons baking powder
- 1 cup coconut sugar
- 1 teaspoon ginger powder
- A pinch of cinnamon powder
- 15 tablespoons coconut butter
- 3 tablespoons maple syrup
- 3 tablespoons flax meal mixed with 3 tablespoons water
- 1 carrot, grated

**Directions:**

1. Grease a heatproof pudding pan with a drizzle of oil.
2. In a blender, mix flour with baking powder, sugar, cinnamon, ginger,

butter, maple syrup and flax meal and pulse well.

3. Add dried fruits and carrot, fold them into the batter and spread this mix into the pudding mold.
4. Put the pudding in your air fryer and cook at 365 degrees F for 30 minutes.
5. Leave the pudding aside to cool down, slice and serve.
6. Enjoy!

### 218. Sweet Strawberry Mix

Servings： 10
Cooking Time: 20 Minutes
**Ingredients:**
- 2 tablespoons lemon juice
- 2 pounds strawberries
- 4 cups coconut sugar
- 1 teaspoon cinnamon powder
- 1 teaspoon vanilla extract

**Directions:**
1. In a pan that fits your air fryer, mix strawberries with coconut sugar, lemon juice, cinnamon and vanilla, stir gently, introduce in the fryer and cook at 350 degrees F for 20 minutes
2. Divide into bowls and serve cold.
3. Enjoy!

### 219. Quinoa Carrot Cake

Servings： 6
Cooking Time: 7 Minutes
**Ingredients:**
- 1½ cups cooked white quinoa
- ½ cup uncooked quinoa
- ¼ cup coconut flour
- ½ cup cooked carrot puree
- 1 cup freshly grated carrots
- 3 tbsp. flaxmeal in 8 tbsp. water (allow to gel for 5 minutes)
- 1 tsp. baking soda
- 1 tsp. baking powder
- 1 tsp. cinnamon
- ½ tsp. nutmeg
- ½ tsp. ground ginger
- 2 tbsp. blackstrap molasses
- Raisins, to taste

**Directions:**
1. Combine all the ingredients at once in a large bowl and mix well. Coat a baking dish with coconut oil and pour in the cake batter.

2. Bake in the air fryer at 350 degrees Fahrenheit for 7 minutes.
3. Once done, let the cake cool and, if desired, frost with vegan cream cheese frosting.

### 220. Simple And Sweet Bananas

Servings： 4
Cooking Time: 15 Minutes
**Ingredients:**
- 3 tablespoons coconut butter
- 2 tablespoons flax meal combined with 2 tablespoons water
- 8 bananas, peeled and halved
- ½ cup corn flour
- 3 tablespoons cinnamon powder
- 1 cup vegan breadcrumbs

**Directions:**
1. Heat up a pan with the butter over medium-high heat, add breadcrumbs, stir and cook for 4 minutes and then transfer to a bowl.
2. Roll each banana in flour, flax meal and breadcrumbs mix.
3. Arrange bananas in your air fryer's basket, dust with cinnamon sugar and cook at 280 degrees F for 10 minutes.
4. Transfer to plates and serve.
5. Enjoy!

### 221. Espresso Vanilla Dessert

Servings: 4
Cooking Time: 20 Minutes
**Ingredients:**
- 1 cup almond milk
- 4 tablespoons flax meal
- 2 tablespoons coconut flour
- 2 and ½ cups water
- 2 tablespoons stevia
- 1 teaspoon espresso powder
- 2 teaspoons vanilla extract
- Coconut cream for serving

**Directions:**
1. In a pan that fits your air fryer, mix flax meal with flour, water, stevia, milk, vanilla and espresso powder, stir, introduce in the fryer and cook at 365 degrees F for 20 minutes.
2. Divide into bowls and serve with coconut cream on top.
3. Enjoy!

### 222. Yogurt Soufflé

Servings: 2
Cooking Time: 14 Minutes
**Ingredients:**
- 1 tbsp unmelted vegan butter
- ¼ cup sugar
- 1 cup dairy free yogurt
- A pinch salt
- ¼ tsp vanilla extract
- 3 tbsp flour
- ½ cup aquafaba
- 3 oz dairy free coconut heavy cream

**Directions:**
1. Coat two 6-oz ramekins with the vegan butter.
2. Pour in the sugar and swirl in the ramekins to coat the butter. Pour out the remaining sugar and reserve.
3. Melt the remaining vegan butter in a microwave and set aside.
4. In a bowl, whisk the butter, yogurt, salt, vanilla extract, flour, and half of the aquafaba. Set aside.
5. In another bowl, beat the remaining aquafaba with the coconut cream until foamy.
6. Fold the coconut cream mixture into the yogurt mix one-third portion at a time as you thoroughly combine.
7. Preheat the air fryer.
8. Share the mix into the ramekins with ½-inch space left on top.
9. Put the ramekins in the fryer basket and bake at 350 F for 14 minutes.
10. When ready, remove and serve.

### 223. Delicious Dried Fruitcake

Servings: 4
Cooking Time: 50 Minutes
**Ingredients:**
- 100 g / 0.22 cup dried apricot
- 50 g / 1.76 oz dried plums
- 40 g / 1.4 oz raisins
- 30 g / 1 oz dried cherries
- 200 g / 0.44 lbs rice flour
- 1/3 cup coconut milk
- 1 teaspoon vanilla sugar
- 1 teaspoon cinnamon
- 2 teaspoon sugar powder

**Directions:**
1. Take the dried apricots and chop it roughly. Then make the same procedure with the plums. Take the big bowl and combine dried and chopped fruits together and add raisins. Stir it and add dried cherries. Take another bowl and combine rice flour, vanilla sugar and cinnamon together in it. Stir it gently and pour the coconut milk in it. Take the hand mixer and mix the mass till it gets smooth. Preheat the oven to 180 C / 360 F. Meanwhile, take the tray and cover it with baking sheet. Transfer dough on it and make it flat. Then put chopped dried fruits on it. Transfer the cake to the air fryer and close the lid. Cook it for 25 minutes. Reduce the heat to the last 5 minutes. Then open the lid and leave the cake for 5 minutes more. Remove it from the air fryer and sprinkle it with sugar powder. Cut it into pieces. Serve it hot.

### 224. Small Batch Brownies

Servings: 4
Cooking Time: 20 Minutes
**Ingredients:**
- For the Dry
- ½ cup whole-wheat, gluten-free pastry flour
- 1 tbsp. ground flax seeds
- ¼ cup cocoa powder
- ½ cup vegan sugar
- ¼ tsp. salt
- Wet Ingredients:
- ¼ cup almond milk
- ½ tsp. pure vanilla extract
- ¼ cup aquafaba
- Extras:
- ¼ cup of: hazelnuts, chopped walnuts, pecans, shredded coconut, mini vegan chocolate chips

**Directions:**
1. Mix all the dry ingredients in one bowl.
2. In a Pyrex jug, mix all the wet and set aside.
3. Add the wet ingredients to the dry and mix to combine.
4. Add in the extra ingredients of your choice and mix again.
5. Preheat the air fryer to 350 degrees Fahrenheit.
6. Line a 5-inch cake tin with baking parchment paper if you want an oil-free

recipe or spray the cake tin lightly with cooking oil spray if the recipe is not oil-free.

7. Place the pan in the air fryer basket.
8. Cook the brownies for 20 minutes. If the brownies are not done cook for 5 minutes more and repeat as needed. A cake tester inserted should come out relatively clean.
9. Recipe Notes:
10. Cooking times may vary depending on the size of the cake tin and the brand of air fryer used.

## 225. No-bake Vegan Strawberry Pie

Servings:4
Cooking Time:5 Minutes
**Ingredients:**
- ½ cup raw cashews
- 8 medjool dates , pitted and roughly chopped
- 1 cup old fashioned rolled oats (use certified gluten-free oats if gluten is a concern)
- 2-3 tablespoons apple juice
- 1 12.3-ounce package Morinu organic firm silken tofu
- 2 medjool dates , pitted and chopped
- 3 tablespoons lemon juice
- 1 tablespoon chia seeds , ground in a blender or coffee mill
- 1 teaspoon grated lemon rind
- 1 vanilla bean (or 1 teaspoon vanilla extract)
- ½ cup apple juice
- 2 teaspoons agar powder (or 2 tablespoons agar flakes)
- stevia , erythritol, or other sweetener to taste
- 12 ounces strawberries , stemmed and sliced

**Directions:**
1. Before You Begin: Place the cashews in a small bowl and add water to cover them by about 1 inch. Set aside to soak for at least 2 hours or in the refrigerator overnight.
2. Crust: Place the 8 chopped dates into a food processor fitted with a metal blade. Add the oats and process until crumbly. With the machine running, add 2 tablespoons of apple juice. Continue to process until mixture begins to adhere together. If necessary, add more juice a teaspoon at a time, but be careful not to add too much. You want it to be sticky but not wet. Press into the bottom of an 8-inch pie pan and up the sides about 1 inch. Set aside.
3. Filling: Drain the cashews and place them in the blender (a Vitamix or other high-speed blender works best, but others should be able to do a good job). Add the tofu, 2 dates, lemon juice, chia seeds, and lemon rind. Split the vanilla bean lengthwise and use a spoon to scrape out the seeds inside; add them to the blender. Blend on high speed until completely smooth, stopping to scrape down the sides to make sure all Ingredients: are incorporated.
4. Taste the filling mixture and add sweetener to taste. (I increased the lemon flavor by using NuNaturals Lemon Stevia.) Leave the mixture in the blender as you continue with the next step.
5. Also, you can do the same with an air fryer just without baking
6. The next steps require you to work quickly. Heat the ½ cup of apple juice in a small sauce pan. As it's heating, sprinkle it with the agar powder. Stir and heat until agar dissolves and juice begins to boil. Cook, stirring, for 1 minute after boiling. Quickly, add the agar mixture to the contents of the blender. Put the top on the blender and blend at high speed until well-blended. Scrape down the sides and blend again briefly. Pour into the prepared crust and smooth the top. Refrigerate until chilled and set.
7. Top with sliced strawberries before serving.

## 226. Plum Cobbler

Servings: 2
Cooking Time: 12 Minutes
**Ingredients:**
- ¼ cup sugar
- ¼ cup flour
- ½ cup cornmeal
- 1 tbsp baking powder
- A pinch of salt

- 4 tbsp melted vegan butter + extra for greasing
- 1 tsp vanilla extract
- 4 tbsp plant milk
- 2 cups stewed plums
- 1 tsp lemon juice

**Directions:**
1. In a bowl, mix the sugar, flour, cornmeal, baking powder, vegan butter, vanilla extract, and milk until smoothly combined.
2. Grease a 3 x 3 baking dish with the remaining butter and pour in the plums with lemon juice. Stir to combine.
3. Spoon the flour mixture on top and use a spoon to level the mix.
4. Place the dish in the fryer basket and bake at 390 F for 12 minutes.
5. Remove after; allow cooling for a few minutes, and serve with vegan ice cream.

### 227. Rose Meringue Kisses

Servings: 4
Cooking Time: 40 Minutes
**Ingredients:**
- ¼ cup aquafaba
- 4 tbsp caster sugar
- ½ tsp rose water
- Pink food coloring

**Directions:**
1. Pour the aquafaba into a bowl and whisk with an electric mixer until a soft peak forms.
2. Gradually, add the sugar while whisking until well-combined. Fold in the rose water and pink food coloring to achieve the intensity of pink color as desired.
3. Spoon the mixture into a piping bag and squeeze out mounds on a cookie sheet that fits into the fryer basket.
4. Preheat the air fryer and bake the meringues at 200 F for 40 minutes or until the meringues are firm like a biscuit.
5. Remove to cool and serve.

### 228. Oatmeal Chocolate Chip Cookies

Servings: 24
Cooking Time:15 minutes
**Ingredients:**
- 1/2 teaspoon of vanilla extract (optional)

- 1/4 tsp of sea salt
- 2 tablespoons of almond butter (use any other vegan seed or nut butter of your choosing)
- 3/4 cup of almond flour (alternatively, use almond meal)
- 1/4 cup of vegan dark chocolate (chopped bar or chips variety)
- 1/4 cup of unsweetened coconut (shredded finely — desiccated; you can try and substitute GF flour blend with oats or almond meal)
- ¼ cup of aquafaba (that is, the liquid or brine found in a can of chickpeas)
- 3/4 cup of rolled oats
- 3 tablespoon of melted coconut oil or avocado oil
- 3/4 teaspoon of baking powder
- 1/3 cup of packed organic brown sugar (alternatively, use muscovado sugar or sub coconut sugar)

**Directions:**
1. Get a large-sized bowl and put in sugar, salt, baking powder, almond flour, coconut vegan chocolate, and oats. Mix together to combine.
2. Get another bowl and pour in the aquafaba. Get a handheld mixer or whisk and beat vigorously until it forms light and fluffy loose peaks. You can introduce a bit of tartar cream to help with the whipping.
3. Add the oil, almond butter, and vanilla (optional) into the aquafaba. Proceed to beat to mix well. Should the mixture look a little deflated, it's all right.
4. Go on to add the mixture to the dry ingredients and mix well to combine. After mixing, a firm, semi-tacky dough should be formed. Cover the dough and store in a refrigerator for between half an hour to overnight.
5. Begin preheating the air fryer to 350 degrees Fahrenheit. Proceed to line the air fryer pan with parchment paper or grease lightly with oil.
6. Start scooping the chilled dough into about 2-tablespoon portions and mold into small discs. Place the discs into the air fryer pan, leaving about an inch worth of gap between the cookies to allow for even heating and spreading.

The amount of cookies that can be cooked at once depends on your air fryer model.

7. Set the timer on the air fryer to bake the cookies for 10 minutes. Go on to increase the temperature of the air fryer to 375 degrees Fahrenheit and bake the cookies for two to four minutes more, or until they turn a shade of golden brown around the edges. Be careful not to burn the cookies, particularly the bottom part as they cook quickly when nearing doneness.
8. Take out the air fryer pan and let the cookies sit for five minutes to cool. Grab a spatula and carefully loosen the cookies as they tend to stick a little while cooking.
9. Store any leftover cookies at room temperature in a loosely sealed container. They can stay good for up to three days in such conditions. When stored in a refrigerator, they can be stored for about four days. In freezers, they can go up to a month. Storing in a freezer immediately after cooking can help the cookies retain their crispy exterior.
10. These cookies are even better when eaten warm or with hot cocoa and almond milk for dipping.

### 229. Orange Cake

Servings： 4
Cooking Time: 30 Minutes
**Ingredients:**
- Cooking spray
- 1 teaspoon baking powder
- 1 cup almond flour
- 1 cup coconut sugar
- ½ teaspoon cinnamon powder
- 3 tablespoons coconut oil, melted
- ½ cup almond milk
- ½ cup pecans, chopped
- ¾ cup water
- ½ cup raisins
- ½ cup orange peel, grated
- ¾ cup orange juice

**Directions:**
1. In a bowl, mix flour with half of the sugar, baking powder, cinnamon, 2

tablespoons oil, milk, pecans and raisins, stir and pour this in a greased cake pan that fits your air fryer.
2. Heat up a small pan over medium heat, add water, orange juice, orange peel, the rest of the oil and the rest of the sugar, stir, bring to a boil, pour over the mix from the pan, introduce in the fryer and cook at 330 degrees F for 30 minutes.
3. Serve cold.
4. Enjoy!

### 230. Cinnamon Pears

Servings： 2-4
Cooking Time: 10 Minutes
**Ingredients:**
- 2 unripe pears, peeled, cored, cut in half
- 2 tbsp. vegan butter
- 1 tsp. pure vanilla extract
- ½ tsp. cinnamon
- To Garnish:
- Sprinkle of nutmeg

**Directions:**
1. Preheat the air fryer to 350 degrees Fahrenheit.
2. Melt the butter and add to it the vanilla extract and cinnamon, mixing well.
3. Baste the cut sides of the pears with the butter and place them cut side down into a baking pan that fits the air fryer.
4. Baste the top of the pears and bake at 350 degrees Fahrenheit for 10 minutes.
5. Flip the pears over and baste again.
6. Bake for 2 more minutes at the same temperature.
7. Give the pears a final baste and set on to serving plates.
8. Serve hot with whipped cream or ice cream.

### 231. Vanilla And Blueberry Squares

Servings： 8
Cooking Time: 20 Minutes
**Ingredients:**
- 5 ounces coconut oil, melted
- ½ teaspoon baking powder
- 4 tablespoons stevia
- 1 teaspoon vanilla
- 4 ounces coconut cream
- 3 tablespoons flax meal combined with 3 tablespoons water

- ½ cup blueberries

**Directions:**
1. In a bowl, mix coconut oil with flax meal, coconut cream, vanilla, stevia and baking powder and blend using an immersion blender.
2. Fold blueberries, pour everything into a square baking dish that fits your air fryer, introduce in the fryer and cook at 320 degrees F for 20 minutes.
3. Slice into squares and serve cold.
4. Enjoy!

### 232. Blackberries Coconut Scones

Servings: 10
Cooking Time: 10 Minutes
**Ingredients:**
- ½ cup coconut flour
- 1 cup blackberries
- 2 tablespoons flax meal combined with 2 tablespoons water
- ½ cup coconut cream
- ½ cup coconut butter
- ½ cup almond flour
- 5 tablespoons stevia
- 2 teaspoons vanilla extract
- 2 teaspoons baking powder

**Directions:**
1. In a bowl, mix almond flour with coconut flour, baking powder and blackberries and stir well.
2. In another bowl, mix cream with butter, vanilla extract, stevia and flax meal and stir well.
3. Combine the 2 mixtures, stir until you obtain your dough, shape 10 triangles from this mix, place them on a lined baking sheet, introduce in the air fryer and cook at 350 degrees F for 10 minutes.
4. Serve them cold.
5. Enjoy!

### 233. Fruit Kebab

Servings: 10
Cooking Time: 6 Minutes
**Ingredients:**
- 1 teaspoon maple syrup
- 1 teaspoon lemon juice
- 1 apple, diced
- 1 mango, diced
- 1 pear, diced

- Salt to taste
- Lemon zest

**Directions:**
1. In a bowl, combine maple syrup and lemon juice.
2. Coat the fruit cubes with the mixture.
3. Season with salt.
4. Arrange in skewers.
5. Place the skewers inside the air fryer and cook at 360 degrees for 5 minutes.
6. Garnish with lemon zest.

### 234. Raspberry Mug Cakes

Servings: 4
Cooking Time: 5 Minutes
**Ingredients:**
- ¼ cup flour
- 1 tsp baking powder
- 5 tbsp sugar
- ½ cup chopped dairy free white chocolate, melted
- 4 tbsp almond milk
- 3 tsp melted vegan butter
- 1 tsp vanilla extract
- A pinch salt
- ½ cup raspberries

**Directions:**
1. In a bowl, mix all the ingredients except the raspberries until properly combined and pour into 4 mugs leaving 1 – inch space on top for rising.
2. Divide the raspberries into the mugs and fold into the mixture.
3. Place 2 cups in the fryer basket and bake at 380 F for 5 minutes or until the cakes set.
4. Remove and cook the remaining batter.
5. Allow cooling and serve.

### 235. Cinnamon Rice

Servings: 4
Cooking Time: 35 Minutes
**Ingredients:**
- 3 and ½ cups water
- 1 cup coconut sugar
- 2 cups white rice, washed and rinsed
- 2 cinnamon sticks
- ½ cup coconut, shredded

**Directions:**
1. In your air fryer, mix water with coconut sugar, rice, cinnamon and

coconut, stir, cover and cook at 365 degrees F for 35 minutes.
2. Divide pudding into cups and serve cold.
3. Enjoy!

### 236. Oatmeal Raisin Cookies

Servings:5
Cooking Time: 7 Minutes Bake: 347°f
**Ingredients:**
- ¼ cup plus ½ tablespoon vegan margarine
- 2½ tablespoons nondairy milk, plain and unsweetened
- ½ cup organic sugar
- ½ teaspoon vanilla extract
- ½ teaspoon plus ⅛ teaspoon ground cinnamon
- ½ cup plus 2 tablespoons flour (whole-wheat pastry, gluten-free all-purpose, or all-purpose)
- ¼ teaspoon sea salt
- ¾ cup rolled oats
- ¼ teaspoon baking soda
- ¼ teaspoon baking powder
- 2 tablespoons raisins
- Cooking oil spray (sunflower, safflower, or refined coconut)

**Directions:**
1. In a medium bowl, using an electric beater, whip the margarine until fluffy.
2. Add in the milk, sugar, and vanilla. Stir or whip with beaters until well combined.
3. In a separate bowl, add the cinnamon, flour, salt, oats, baking soda, and baking powder and stir well to combine. Add the dry mixture to the wet mixture and combine everything well with a wooden spoon. Stir in the raisins.
4. Preheat the air fryer basket (with your 6-inch round, 2-inch deep baking pan inside) for 2 minutes. Then, spray the pan lightly with oil. Drop tablespoonfuls of the batter onto the pan, leaving a little room in between each one as they'll probably spread out a bit. Bake for about 7 minutes, or until lightly browned.
5. Gently transfer to a cooling rack (or plate), being careful to leave the cookies intact. Repeat as desired, making all of the cookies at once, or

keeping the batter on hand in the fridge to be used later (it will keep refrigerated in an airtight container for a week to 10 days).

### 237. Apple Cinnamon Scuffins

Servings: 4
Cooking Time: 15 Minutes
**Ingredients:**
- 2 cups oat flour
- 1 tsp baking powder
- 1 cup rolled oats
- ½ tsp baking soda
- ¼ tsp salt
- 1 tsp cinnamon powder
- ½ cup date paste
- ½ cup currants
- ½ cup dairy free yogurt
- ½ cup almond milk
- ½ cups chopped red apples
- Confectioner's sugar for sprinkling

**Directions:**
1. In a bowl, combine all the dry ingredients. Then, in another bowl, mix the date paste, dairy-free yogurt, and almond milk.
2. Add the cinnamon mixture to the milk mixture and combine. After, fold in the apples.
3. In a baking sheet that can fit into the air fryer, line with parchment paper, and drop large spoonfuls of the batter on the sheet.
4. Sprinkle with confectioner's sugar and bake at 350 F for 12 to 15 minutes.
5. Remove when ready, allow cooling, and serve.

### 238. Dates And Cashew Sticks

Servings: 6
Cooking Time: 15 Minutes
**Ingredients:**
- 1/3 cup stevia
- ¼ cup almond meal
- 1 tablespoon almond butter
- 1 and ½ cups cashews, chopped
- 4 dates, chopped
- ¾ cup coconut, shredded
- 1 tablespoon chia seeds

**Directions:**

1. In a bowl, mix stevia with almond meal, almond butter, cashews, coconut, dates and chia seeds and stir well again.
2. Spread this on a lined baking sheet that fits your air fryer, press well, introduce in the fryer and cook at 300 degrees F for 15 minutes.
3. Leave mix to cool down, cut into medium sticks and serve.
4. Enjoy!

## 239. Chocolate Chip Cookies

Servings:6
Cooking Time: 7 Minutes Bake: 347°f
**Ingredients:**
- 1 tablespoon refined coconut oil, melted
- 1 tablespoon maple syrup
- 1 tablespoon nondairy milk
- ½ teaspoon vanilla
- ¼ cup plus 2 tablespoons whole-wheat pastry flour or all-purpose gluten-free flour
- 2 tablespoons coconut sugar
- ¼ teaspoon sea salt
- ¼ teaspoon baking powder
- 2 tablespoons vegan chocolate chips
- Cooking oil spray (sunflower, safflower, or refined coconut)

**Directions:**
1. In a medium bowl, stir together the oil, maple syrup, milk, and vanilla. Add the flour, coconut sugar, salt, and baking powder. Stir just until thoroughly combined. Stir in the chocolate chips.
2. Preheat the air fryer basket (with a 6-inch round, 2-inch deep baking pan inside) for 2 minutes. Then, spray the pan lightly with oil. Drop tablespoonfuls of the batter onto the pan, leaving a little room in between in case they spread out a bit. Bake for 7 minutes, or until lightly browned. Be careful not to overcook.
3. Gently transfer to a cooling rack (or plate). Repeat as desired, making all of the cookies at once, or keeping the batter on hand in the fridge to be used later (it will keep refrigerated in an airtight container for about a week). Enjoy warm if possible!

## 240. Berry Crumble

Servings:   4
Cooking Time: 12 Minutes
**Ingredients:**
- ½ cup blackberries
- ½ cup strawberries
- 1 cup blueberries
- ¼ cup flour
- ¼ cup sugar
- 1 teaspoon vanilla
- ½ cup quick oats
- ¼ cup brown sugar
- 1 teaspoon lemon juice
- 3 tablespoons melted butter

**Directions:**
1. In a bowl, combine the berries, lemon juice and sugar.
2. In another bowl, mix the rest of the ingredients.
3. Toss the berries in the mixture.
4. Spray air fryer with oil.
5. Cook at 390 degrees F for 12 minutes.

## 241. Oatmeal Pudding

Servings: 4
Cooking Time: 55 Minutes
**Ingredients:**
- 200 g / 0.44 lbs oatmeal
- 100 g / 0.4 cup soy milk
- 100 g / 0.22 lbs rice
- 50 g / 0.2 cup almond milk
- 10 g / 0.35 oz wheat
- 1 teaspoon cinnamon
- 1 teaspoon flour
- 1 teaspoon lemon zest
- 1 apple

**Directions:**
1. Take the oatmeal and put it in the big bowl. Then add rice, cinnamon, and flour. Peel the apple and grate it. Add grated apple to the dry mixture and stir it carefully. Then add lemon zest and wheat. Stir it gently. Pour the mass into the soy milk and almond milk. Stir it carefully and leave it for 10 minutes. Meanwhile, preheat the air fryer to 200 C / 390 F and transfer the pudding to it. Reduce the temperature to 320 F and cook it for 20 minutes. Remove the pudding from the air fryer and chill it

little. The pudding should be warm but not hot. Serve it immediately. Enjoy!

## 242. Cinnamon Bananas

Servings: 4
Cooking Time: 15 Minutes
**Ingredients:**
- 3 tablespoons coconut butter
- 2 tablespoons flax meal combined with 2 tablespoons water
- 8 bananas, peeled and halved
- ½ cup corn flour
- 3 tablespoons cinnamon powder
- 1 cup vegan breadcrumbs

**Directions:**
1. Heat up a pan with the butter over medium-high heat, add breadcrumbs, stir and cook for 4 minutes and then transfer to a bowl.
2. Roll each banana in flour, flax meal and breadcrumbs mix.
3. Arrange bananas in your air fryer's basket, dust with cinnamon sugar and cook at 280 degrees F for 10 minutes.
4. Transfer to plates and serve.
5. Enjoy!

## 243. Easy Pumpkin Cake

Servings: 10
Cooking Time: 40 Minutes
**Ingredients:**
- 1 and ½ teaspoons baking powder
- Cooking spray
- 1 cup pumpkin puree
- 2 cups almond flour
- ½ teaspoon baking soda
- 1 and ½ teaspoons cinnamon, ground
- ¼ teaspoon ginger, ground
- 1 tablespoon coconut oil, melted
- 1 tablespoon flaxseed mixed with 2 tablespoons water
- 1 tablespoon vanilla extract
- 1/3 cup maple syrup
- 1 teaspoon lemon juice

**Directions:**
1. In a bowl, flour with baking powder, baking soda, cinnamon and ginger and stir.
2. Add flaxseed, coconut oil, vanilla, pumpkin puree, maple syrup and lemon juice, stir and pour into a greased cake pan.

3. Introduce in your air fryer, cook at 330 degrees F for 40 minutes, leave aside to cool down, slice and serve.
4. Enjoy!

## 244. Blueberry Apple Crumble

Servings: 2
Cooking Time: 15 Minutes
**Ingredients:**
- 1 apple, finely diced
- ¼ cup brown rice flour plus 1 tbsp. more
- ½ cup frozen strawberries, blueberries or peaches
- 2 tbsp. nondairy butter
- 2 tbsp. sugar
- ½ tsp. ground cinnamon

**Directions:**
1. Preheat the air fryer to 350 degrees Fahrenheit for 5 minutes.
2. Combine the apple and frozen berries or peaches in an air fryer–safe baking pan.
3. In a small bowl, combine the flour, cinnamon, sugar, and butter.
4. Spoon the crumble mixture over the fruit. Sprinkle a little extra flour all the fruit to cover any that are exposed.
5. Cook at 350 degrees Fahrenheit for 15 minutes.
6. Serve warm with dairy-free whipped cream or ice cream

## 245. Lemon Cream

Servings: 6
Cooking Time: 30 Minutes
**Ingredients:**
- 1 and 1/3 pint almond milk
- 1 medium banana
- 4 tablespoons lemon zest, grated
- 3 tablespoons flax meal combined with 3 tablespoons water
- 5 tablespoons stevia
- 2 tablespoons lemon juice

**Directions:**
1. In a bowl, mix mashed banana with milk and swerve and stir very well.
2. Add lemon zest and lemon juice, whisk well, pour into ramekins, place them in your air fryer, cook at 360 degrees F for 30 minutes and serve cold.
3. Enjoy!

## 246. Grape Pudding

Servings: 6
Cooking Time: 40 Minutes
**Ingredients:**
- 1 cup grapes curd
- 3 cups grapes
- 3 and ½ ounces maple syrup
- 3 tablespoons flax meal combined with 3 tablespoons water
- 2 ounces coconut butter, melted
- 3 and ½ ounces almond milk
- ½ cup almond flour
- ½ teaspoon baking powder

**Directions:**
1. In a bowl, mix the half of the fruit curd with the grapes stir and divide into 6 heatproof ramekins.
2. In a bowl, mix flax meal with maple syrup, melted coconut butter, the rest of the curd, baking powder, milk and flour and stir well.
3. Divide this into the ramekins as well, introduce in the fryer and cook at 200 degrees F for 40 minutes.
4. Leave puddings to cool down and serve!
5. Enjoy!

## 247. Easy Cinnamon Crisps

Servings:4
Cooking Time: 5 To 6 Minutes Fry: 347°f
**Ingredients:**
- 1 (8-inch) tortilla, preferably sprouted whole-grain
- Cooking oil spray (sunflower, safflower, or refined coconut)
- 2 teaspoons coconut sugar
- ½ teaspoon cinnamon

**Directions:**
1. Cut the tortilla into 8 triangles (like a pizza). Place on a large plate and spray both sides with oil.
2. Sprinkle the tops evenly with the coconut sugar and cinnamon. In short spurts, spray the tops again with the oil. (If you spray too hard for this step, it will make the powdery toppings fly off!)
3. Place directly in the air fryer basket in a single layer (it's okay if they overlap a little, but do your best to give them space). Fry for 5 to 6 minutes, or until the triangles are lightly browned, but

not too brown—they're bitter if overcooked. Enjoy warm if possible.

## 248. Strawberry Puffs With Creamy Lemon Sauce

Servings:8
Cooking Time: 10 Minutes Bake: 320°f
**Ingredients:**
- For the filling
- 3 cups sliced strawberries, fresh or frozen (1½ pints or 24 ounces)
- 1 cup sugar-free strawberry jam (sweetened only with fruit juice)
- 1 tablespoon arrowroot (or cornstarch)
- Cooking oil spray (sunflower, safflower, or refined coconut)
- 8 large (13-inch x 17-inch) sheets of phyllo dough, thawed (see Ingredient Tip)
- For the sauce
- 1 cup raw cashew pieces (see Cooking Tip)
- ¼ cup plus 2 tablespoons raw agave nectar
- ¼ cup plus 1 tablespoon water
- 3 tablespoons fresh lemon juice
- 2 teaspoons (packed) lemon zest (see Cooking Tip)
- 2 tablespoons neutral-flavored oil (sunflower, safflower, or refined coconut)
- 2 teaspoons vanilla
- ¼ teaspoon sea salt

**Directions:**
1. In a medium bowl, add the strawberries, jam, and arrowroot and stir well to combine. Set aside.
2. Spray the air fryer basket with oil and set aside.
3. To assemble the puffs
4. Gently unwrap the phyllo dough. Remove 8 sheets and carefully set them aside. Re-wrap the remaining phyllo in airtight plastic wrap and place back in the fridge.
5. Remove 1 large sheet of phyllo and place on a clean, dry surface. Spray with the oil. Fold it into thirds so that it forms a long, skinny rectangle. As you go, spray each portion of dry phyllo, so the exposed phyllo continually gets lightly coated with oil.

6. Place about ⅓ cup of the strawberry mixture at the base of the phyllo rectangle. Fold the bottom of the phyllo up and over the mixture. Continue to fold up toward the top, forming it into a triangle as you go. Once fully wrapped, place it in the air fryer basket and spray the top with oil.
7. Repeat with the remaining phyllo and strawberry mixture. Note you'll probably only be able to fit 3 puffs in your air fryer at a time, because you don't want them to overlap.
8. Bake for 10 minutes, or until beautifully golden-browned.
9. To make the sauce
10. Place the cashews, agave, water, lemon juice and zest, oil, vanilla, and salt in a blender. Process until completely smooth and velvety. (Any leftover sauce will keep nicely in the fridge for up to a week.)
11. Transfer the strawberry puffs to a plate and drizzle with the creamy lemon sauce. If desired, garnish with sliced strawberries. Enjoy while warm.

## 249. Apple Cake

Servings: 6
Cooking Time: 40 Minutes
**Ingredients:**
- 3 cups apples, cored and cubed
- 1 cup coconut sugar
- 1 tablespoon vanilla extract
- 2 tablespoons flax meal combined with 3 tablespoons water
- 1 tablespoon apple pie spice
- 2 cups whole wheat flour
- 1 tablespoon baking powder
- 2 tablespoons vegetable oil

**Directions:**
1. In a bowl mix flax meal with oil, apple pie spice, apples, vanilla and sugar and stir using your mixer
2. In another bowl, mix baking powder with flour and stir.
3. Combine the 2 mixtures, stir and pour into a springform pan.
4. Put springform pan in your air fryer and cook at 320 degrees F for 40 minutes
5. Slice and serve.
6. Enjoy!

## 250. Cocoa Brownies

Servings:  12
Cooking Time: 20 Minutes
**Ingredients:**
- 6 ounces coconut oil, melted
- 3 tablespoons flax meal combined with 3 tablespoons water
- 3 ounces cocoa powder
- 2 teaspoons vanilla
- ½ teaspoon baking powder
- 4 ounces coconut cream
- 5 tablespoons stevia

**Directions:**
1. In a blender, mix flax meal with oil, cocoa powder, baking powder, vanilla, cream and stevia and stir using a mixer.
2. Pour this into a lined baking dish that fits your air fryer, introduce in the fryer and cook at 350 degrees F for 20 minutes.
3. Slice into rectangles and serve cold
4. Enjoy!

## 251. Gooey Lemon Bars

Servings:6
Cooking Time: 25 Minutes Bake: 347°f
**Ingredients:**
- For the crust
- ¾ cup whole-wheat pastry flour
- 2 tablespoons powdered sugar
- ¼ cup refined coconut oil, melted
- For the filling
- ½ cup organic sugar
- 1 packed tablespoon lemon zest (see Cooking Tip)
- ¼ cup fresh lemon juice
- ⅛ teaspoon sea salt
- ¼ cup unsweetened, plain applesauce
- 1¾ teaspoons arrowroot (or cornstarch)
- ¾ teaspoon baking powder
- Cooking oil spray (sunflower, safflower, or refined coconut)

**Directions:**
1. Spray a 6-inch round, 2-inch deep baking pan lightly with oil. Remove the crust mixture from the fridge and gently press it into the bottom of the pan to form a crust. Place in the air fryer and bake for 5 minutes, or until it becomes slightly firm to the touch.

2. Remove and spread the lemon filling over the crust. Bake for about 18 to 20 minutes, or until the top is nicely browned. Remove and allow to cool for an hour or more in the fridge. Once firm and cooled, cut into pieces and serve. You might use a fork to get each piece out, as the pan is a little small for traditional spatulas.

## 252. Cauliflower Pudding

Servings: 4
Cooking Time: 30 Minutes
**Ingredients:**
- 2 and ½ cups water
- 1 cup coconut sugar
- 2 cups cauliflower rice
- 2 cinnamon sticks
- ½ cup coconut, shredded

**Directions:**
1. In a pan that fits your air fryer, mix water with coconut sugar, cauliflower rice, cinnamon and coconut, stir, introduce in the fryer and cook at 365 degrees F for 30 minutes
2. Divide pudding into cups and serve cold.
3. Enjoy!

## 253. Strawberry Lemonade Pop Tart

Servings: 14
Cooking Time: 10 Minutes
**Ingredients:**
- For the Strawberry Chia Jam:
- 3 cups sliced strawberries, frozen or fresh
- 3 tbsp. chia seeds
- 2 tsp. maple syrup, or to taste
- 2 tbsp. lemon juice, or to taste
- For the Pop-tarts:
- 1 cup all-purpose flour
- 1 cup whole-wheat pastry flour
- 2 tbsp. light brown sugar
- ¼ tsp. salt
- ½ cup ice cold water
- ⅔ cup very cold coconut oil
- ½ tsp. vanilla extract
- For the Lemon Glaze:
- 1¼ cup powdered sugar
- Zest of 1 lemon
- 2 tbsp. lemon juice
- ¼ tsp. vanilla extract
- 1 tsp. melted coconut oil
- Colorful sprinkles for decoration

**Directions:**
1. To make the Chia Jam:
2. In a sauce pan, heat the strawberries and cherries until they start to get syrupy and give out their juice.
3. Once they are super soft, mash them until the mixture is jammy, and still with some visible bits of fruit.
4. Add in the maple syrup and lemon juice Adjust the lemon and maple syrup depending on the level of sweetness in the fruit.
5. Take the mixture off the heat, transfer it to a glass container and add in the chia seeds.
6. Allow the mixture to set for 20 minutes. It will thicken on standing.
7. To make the Pop-tarts:
8. In a large bowl, mix both flours, sugar and salt.
9. Cut in the cold coconut oil with a fork or pastry cutter until the mixture resembles tiny peas.
10. Add the vanilla extract and slowly add in the ice cold water.
11. It should be moist enough to form it into a ball without flaking away, but not too sticky either.
12. Cut the dough in half and flour a work surface and rolling pin.
13. Roll out the dough to just a few millimeters thick then cut into 7 cm by 5 cm rectangles.
14. Place the rectangles on a baking sheet lined with a silicone baking sheet or parchment paper.
15. Place a heaping teaspoon of jam onto half of the dough rectangles. Moisten all around the perimeter of the dough.
16. Top with another dough rectangle, and crimp the edges with a fork to seal.
17. Poke three sets of three holes into the top of the pop tart with your fork. Place pop tarts on the baking sheet in the fridge to set for 20 minutes.
18. Heat the air fryer to 400 degrees Fahrenheit.
19. Add four pop-tarts to the air fryer basket and cook for 10 minutes.

20. Remove and repeat with the remaining pop-tarts until they're all cooked. Cool for 20 minutes before serving.
21. To make the Lemon Glaze:
22. In a bowl, mix together the icing sugar, lemon juice, coconut oil, vanilla extract and lemon zest.
23. Drizzle the icing on each of the pop-tarts and decorate with sprinkles. Let the icing set and enjoy!

### 254. Sweet Cauliflower Rice With Cherries

Servings: 4
Cooking Time: 30 Minutes
**Ingredients:**
- 1 and ½ cups cauliflower rice
- 1 and ½ teaspoons cinnamon powder
- 1/3 cup stevia
- 2 tablespoons coconut butter, melted
- 2 apples, peeled, cored and sliced
- 1 cup natural apple juice
- 3 cups almond milk
- ½ cup cherries, dried

**Directions:**
1. In a pan that fits your air fryer, combine rice with cinnamon, stevia, butter, apples, apple juice, almond milk and cherries, toss, introduce in your air fryer and cook at 365 degrees F for 30 minutes.
2. Divide between bowls and serve.
3. Enjoy!

### 255. Orange Bread With Almonds

Servings: 8
Cooking Time: 40 Minutes
**Ingredients:**
- 1 orange, peeled and sliced
- Juice of 2 oranges
- 3 tablespoons vegetable oil
- 2 tablespoons flax meal combined with 2 tablespoons water
- ¾ cup coconut sugar+ 2 tablespoons
- ¾ cup whole wheat flour
- ¾ cup almonds, ground

**Directions:**
1. Grease a loaf pan with some oil, sprinkle 2 tablespoons sugar and arrange orange slices on the bottom.
2. In a bowl, mix the oil with ¾ cup sugar, almonds, flour and orange juice, stir, spoon this over orange slices, place the

pan in your air fryer and cook at 360 degrees F for 40 minutes.
3. Slice and serve the bread right away.
4. Enjoy!

## Other Vegan Air Fryer Recipes

### 256. Baked Eggplant's Halves

Servings: 4
Cooking Time: 40 Minutes
**Ingredients:**
- 4 eggplants
- 2 yellow onions
- 100 g / 0.4 cup soy milk
- 1 carrot
- 200 g / 0.44 lbs tofu
- 1 teaspoon olive oil
- 100 g / 0.22 lbs soy cheese
- 1 teaspoon black pepper
- 1 teaspoon basil
- 1 teaspoon oregano
- 50 g / 1.76 oz parsley
- 50 g / 0.2 cup water
- 1 teaspoon salt

**Directions:**
1. Wash the eggplants and cut it into 2 parts. Then rub it with salt and leave it. Meanwhile, peel the yellow onions and chop it. Peel the carrot and grate it. Combine chopped the onion and grated carrot together. Sprinkle it with black pepper, basil, oregano and stir it carefully. Take the eggplants and remove the meat from it. Chop the meat and combine it with carrot and onion. Stir it. Chop the parsley and add it to the mixture too. Stir it again. Grate the tofu cheese. Preheat, the air fryer to 190 C / 380 F. Pour the soy milk and water to the air fryer and stir it with the help of a wooden spoon. Fill the eggplants with the vegetable mass and sprinkle each half with grated tofu cheese. Transfer all eggplant's halves to the air fryer and close the lid. Cook it for 20 minutes. Then remove the dish from the air fryer and chill it little. Enjoy!

### 257. Air Fryer Healthy Zucchini Corn Fritters

Servings: 4
Cooking Time: 12 Minutes
**Ingredients:**
- 1 large zucchini
- 1 cup corn kernels
- 1 medium potato cooked
- 2 tbsp plain flour
- 2-3 garlic cloves, minced
- 1-2 tsp olive oil
- Salt and ground black pepper to taste

**Directions:**
1. Grate zucchini using a grater or food processor. Transfer to a large mixing bowl. Season with salt and set aside for 10-15 min. Then squeeze out excess water from the zucchini using clean hands or using a cheesecloth.
2. Grate or mash the cooked potato.
3. Combine zucchini, potato, corn, chickpea flour, garlic, salt and pepper in a mixing bowl.
4. Take nearly 2 tbsp batter, give it a shape of a patty and place them on parchment paper.
5. Lightly brush oil on the surface of each fritter.
6. Preheat air fryer to 360 F.
7. Place the fritters on the preheated air fryer mesh without touching each other. Cook them for 8 min.
8. Then turn the fritters and cook for another 3-4 minute or until well done.
9. Serve warm with ketchup or another dipping sauce you prefer.

### 258. Air Fryer Vegetable Kebabs

Servings: 3
Cooking Time: 10 Minutes
**Ingredients:**
- 2 large bell peppers, cut in large pieces
- 1 medium-sized eggplant
- 1 medium-sized zucchini
- 1 small onion
- Salt and pepper to taste
- 1 tbsp olive oil
- 6-inch skewers

**Directions:**
1. If you're going to use wooden skewers, place them in water for 10 minutes before using.
2. Cut all the veggies in about 1 inch pieces. Thread them on skewers. Drizzle with olive oil and sprinkle with some salt and pepper.
3. Preheat the air fryer to 390 F. Add skewers to the fryer and cook for nearly 10 minutes.
4. Serve and enjoy.

### 259. Air Fryer Bbq Lentil Meatballs

Servings: 5
Cooking Time: 45 Minutes
**Ingredients:**
- 2 cups vegetable broth
- 1 cup dry green or brown lentils
- 1/2 cup dried mushrooms, finely chopped
- 2 tbsp avocado or sesame oil
- 1 large onion, diced
- 1 tbsp tomato paste
- 1 clove garlic, minced
- 1/2 cup vital wheat gluten
- 3 tbsp vegan BBQ sauce
- 2 tbsp water or vegetable broth
- 1 tbsp vegan Worcestershire sauce or low-sodium soy sauce
- 1 tsp onion powder
- 1 tsp dried parsley
- 1/2 tsp smoked paprika
- A pinch of salt to taste
- 1/4 tsp ground black pepper

**Directions:**
1. In a large pot, heated over medium-high, bring the vegetable broth, lentils, and mushrooms to a boil. Adjust heat to medium-low, and simmer for 20 minutes, or until lentils are tender and liquid is absorbed.
2. Meanwhile, in a small sauté pan, warm the oil over medium heat. Once hot, add onions to pan and sauté until onions are caramelizing. Then adjust heat to medium-low, and add tomato paste and garlic to pan. Sauté for another minute, then set the pan aside.
3. In a food processor, place cooked lentil/mushroom mixture, onion/tomato mixture, vital wheat gluten, 3 tablespoons BBQ sauce, water, Worcestershire sauce, onion powder, parsley, smoked paprika, salt, and pepper. Pulse until the mixture is combined, but still chunky (you don't want a chewy hummus!).
4. Preheat the air fryer to 350 F. Lightly spray the basket with cooking oil. Moisten your hands with water, then form roughly 2-tablespoon-sized balls with the lentil mixture. Place each ball in the air fryer basket, leaving at least 1/2-inch between them. Sprinkle balls with oil and cook for nearly 10-12 minutes until golden.
5. Transfer lentil meatballs to a plate and drizzle 1 cup of BBQ sauce over the top.
6. Serve with toothpicks and enjoy!

### 260. Lemony Green Beans

Servings: 4
Cooking Time: 10-12 Minutes
**Ingredients:**
- 1 lemon
- 1 pound green beans, washed and then destem
- 1/4 teaspoon oil
- Black pepper, to taste
- Pinch salt
- Toasted nuts of choice, optional

**Directions:**
1. Except for the nuts, if using, toss the green beans with the rest of the ingredients. Transfer to the air fryer basket.
2. Set the temperature to 400F and set the timer for 10 to 12 minutes.
3. Sprinkle with nuts, if preferred. Serve.

### 261. Asian Spicy Sweet Sauce

Servings:4
Cooking Time: 3 To 5 Minutes
**Ingredients:**
- 2 teaspoons arrowroot (or cornstarch)
- ½ cup water, divided
- ¼ cup tamari or shoyu
- ¼ cup agave nectar
- 1 tablespoon toasted sesame oil
- 4 large garlic cloves, minced or pressed
- ¼ to ½ teaspoon red chili flakes (adjust according to your heat preference)

**Directions:**
1. In a medium pan, whisk the arrowroot with 1 tablespoon of the water until dissolved.
2. Add the remaining water, tamari, agave, sesame oil, garlic, and chili flakes and whisk over medium heat. Continue to cook, whisking often, until it becomes thicker in consistency.
3. Remove from heat when lightly thickened. This will keep, refrigerated in an airtight container, for at least 2 weeks.

### 262. Vegan Air Fryer Bagel Pizzas

Servings: 1
Cooking Time: 5 Minutes
**Ingredients:**
- 1 bagel
- 2 tbsp marinara sauce, divided
- 6 slices vegan pepperoni
- 2 tbsp non-dairy mozzarella cheese, sliced
- A pinch of finely chopped fresh basil

**Directions:**
1. Cut bagel in half.
2. Preheat the air fryer to 370 F and toast bagel halves in air fryer for 2 minutes.
3. Remove bagel halves from the air fryer. Top each half of a bagel with a tablespoon of marinara, three vegan pepperoni slices, and a tablespoon of non-dairy cheese.
4. Return bagel halves to the air fryer basket. Air fry at 370 degrees for 4 to 5 minutes or until the cheese is melted enough.
5. Carefully remove bagel halves from air fryer. Top each bagel pizza with a pinch of chopped fresh basil. The pizzas will be quite hot. So wait a couple of minutes before eating.

### 263. Zucchini Fried Chips

Servings: 3
Cooking Time: 10 Minutes
**Ingredients:**
- 1 large zucchini, sliced according to your preference
- 1 large egg
- ½ cup breadcrumbs
- 1 tsp Italian seasoning
- ¾ tsp garlic salt
- Ground pepper to taste
- 2 tbsp olive oil

**Directions:**
1. Prepare the zucchini for cooking. Slice it into strips or into thin discs. Toss in salt and let it sit for 30 minutes to remove the excess moisture. Rinse with cold water and then pat dry with paper towels.
2. Prepare the ingredients. Whisk the egg in a bowl, add bread crumbs, and Italian seasoning into another. These will serve as your breading.

3. Cover each slice with the breading by first dipping into the egg bath and then on the breadcrumbs mix.
4. Preheat air fryer to 390 F. Place the zucchini slices inside. Cook for about 10 minutes or until crispy.
5. Serve with your dip of choice.

### 264. Savory Zucchini Fries

Servings: 3-4
Cooking Time: 15 Minutes
**Ingredients:**
- 2 large zucchinis cut into 1/2 inch x 3 inch matchsticks
- 1/2 cup all purpose flour
- 1/4 cup aquafaba
- 1 cup Panko breadcrumbs
- 3/4 teaspoon garlic salt
- Ground black pepper to taste

**Directions:**
1. Place flour, aquafaba, and breadcrumbs in three shallow bowls.
2. Cut zucchini into matchsticks.
3. Dip zucchini firstly in flour, then aquafaba, and then into breadcrumbs.
4. Preheat the air fryer to 390 F. Working in batches fry covered zucchini matchsticks for 5-7 minutes, shaking couple times while cooking. Cook until crispy.
5. Serve with dipping sauce you prefer.

### 265. Vegetarian Quesadilla With Black Beans And Sweet Potato

Servings: 4
Cooking Time: 15 Minutes
**Ingredients:**
- 4 medium flour tortillas
- 1 large sweet potato
- 2 large avocados
- 1/2 cup black beans
- 1/4 cup corn
- 1 small red pepper
- 1 small orange pepper
- 1 tbsp taco seasoning
- 1 cup cheddar (optional)
- 2 tsp olive or sesame oil, divided
- Salt and pepper to taste

**Directions:**
1. Using a fork poke several holes into the sweet potato and drizzle with 1 tsp olive oil. Season with a small amount of salt

and pepper. Wrap the sweet potato in paper towels and microwave for 8 minutes or until very tender.

2. Dice peppers removing the ribs and seeds. Add diced peppers to a large pan and cook until tender, about 5-7 minutes. Then add black beans, corn and taco seasoning and stir to combine cooking another 3 minutes. Transfer to a bowl and set aside.

3. Spread about 3 tbsp of sweet potato over the tortilla. Next mash half of an avocado over the sweet potato. Add about 1/4 cup of the veggie/bean filling over the top of the avocado. Finally sprinkle a generous amount of cheese over top (optional).

4. Preheat the air fryer to 370 F. Place the tortilla down on the frying basket and cook for 10-15 minutes until tortilla is browned and cheese is melted. Carefully flip tortilla in half on to itself using the spatula. Repeat until all tortillas are filled and cooked. Slice and serve warm and enjoy!

## 266. Crispy Potato Chips

Servings: 2
Cooking Time: 15 Minutes
**Ingredients:**
- 1 pound Russet Potato, very thinly sliced
- Grapeseed Oil Cooking Spray
- Sea Salt to taste

**Directions:**
1. Slice potatoes very thinly using vegetable slicer. Then use a paper towel to press out as much of the moisture from the potatoes slices as possible.
2. Preheat the air fryer to 450 F. Spray the mesh basket of your air fryer with the oil spray and place the potatoes in a single layer inside. You will have to do this in batches.
3. Spray the tops of the potatoes with the oil spray and sprinkle with salt.
4. Cook until potatoes golden and crisp for about 10-15 minutes depending on potato thickness.
5. Remove the chips from the air fryer and serve them with sauce you like.

## 267. Crunchy Onion Rings

Servings:3
Cooking Time: 14 Minutes Fry: 392°f
**Ingredients:**
- ½ medium-large white onion, peeled
- ½ cup nondairy milk, plain and unsweetened
- ¾ cup flour (whole-wheat pastry, chickpea, or all-purpose gluten-free)
- 1 tablespoon arrowroot (or cornstarch)
- ¾ teaspoon sea salt, divided
- ¾ teaspoon freshly ground black pepper, divided
- ¾ teaspoon garlic granules, divided
- 1 cup bread crumbs (whole grain or gluten-free; see Cooking Tip)
- Cooking oil spray (coconut, sunflower, or safflower)

**Directions:**
1. Cut the onion into thick, ½- to ¾-inch slices. You should have about one cup of onion slices. Carefully separate the onion slices into rings—a gentle touch is important here.
2. Place the milk in a shallow bowl and set aside.
3. Make the first breading. In a medium bowl, combine the flour, arrowroot, ¼ teaspoon salt, ¼ teaspoon pepper, and ¼ teaspoon garlic. Stir well and set aside.
4. Make the second breading. In a separate medium bowl, combine the breadcrumbs with ½ teaspoon salt, ½ teaspoon garlic, and ½ teaspoon onion. Stir well and set aside.
5. Spray the air fryer basket with oil and set aside.
6. Get ready to assemble! Here's how each onion ring will go: Dip one ring into the milk. Then, dip into the flour mixture. Next, dip into the milk again, and back into the flour mixture, coating thoroughly. Dip into the milk one last time, and then dip into the breadcrumb mixture, coating thoroughly. Gently place in the air fryer basket.
7. Repeat with all of the remaining onion rings, gently laying them in the air fryer basket without overlapping too much. Your fingers will get really goopy toward the end of this process. The

good news? You'll make it through, and you can smoosh the coating onto the last pieces once things get a bit messy.

8. Once all of the onion rings are in the air fryer basket, spray the tops generously with the oil spray and fry for 4 minutes. Remove the air fryer basket, spray generously with oil again, and fry for 3 minutes.

9. Remove the air fryer basket and spray the onion rings with oil again. Then oh-so-gently remove and turn the pieces over, so that they cook evenly. Spray generously with oil again and fry for 4 minutes. Remove, spray generously with oil one last time, and cook for 3 minutes, or until the onion rings are very crunchy and browned. Remove carefully and serve with ketchup or another sauce of your choice.

### 268. Crisp Banana Chips

Servings: 2
Cooking Time: 7-8 Minutes
**Ingredients:**
- 1 large-sized plantain banana
- 1 teaspoon coconut oil
- 1/2 teaspoon salt
- 1/4 teaspoon turmeric powder
- Pinch chili powder

**Directions:**
1. Preheat the air fryer to 190C.
2. Peel the plantain and cut it into thin round pieces - do not slice them into wafer thin pieces, otherwise, the chips will fly into the coils when they begin to get crispy.
3. Put the plantain slices into a bowl and toss with the turmeric powder and coconut oil. Transfer to the air fryer basket and set the timer for 7 to 8 minutes, removing and shaking the basket every 2 minutes.
4. The chips are done when they are crisp and light golden brown.
5. When the chips are cooked, let them cool 2 minutes or more to allow them to get crisper. Serve!

### 269. Tamari Roasted Eggplant

Servings: 4
Cooking Time: 13 Minutes Roast: 392°f
**Ingredients:**

- Cooking oil spray (sunflower, safflower, or refined coconut)
- 1 medium-size eggplant (1 pound), cut into ½-inch-thick slices
- 2½ tablespoons tamari or shoyu
- 2 teaspoons garlic granules
- 2 teaspoons onion granules
- 4 teaspoons oil (olive, sunflower, or safflower)

**Directions:**
1. Spray the air fryer basket with oil and set aside.
2. Place the eggplant slices in a large bowl and sprinkle the tamari, garlic, onion, and oil on top. Stir well, coating the eggplant as evenly as possible.
3. Place the eggplant in a single (or at most, double) layer in the air fryer basket. You may need to do this recipe in batches, depending on the size of your air fryer. Set the bowl aside without discarding the liquid.
4. Roast for 5 minutes. Remove and place the eggplant in the bowl again. Toss the eggplant slices to coat evenly with the remaining liquid mixture, and place back in the air fryer as before. Roast for another 3 minutes. Remove the basket and flip the pieces over to ensure even cooking.
5. Roast for another 5 minutes, or until the eggplant is nicely browned and very tender.

### 270. Lentil Cutlets

Servings: 6
Cooking Time: 25 Minutes
**Ingredients:**
- 300 g / 0.66 lbs cooked lentil
- 1 onion
- 1 carrot
- 100 g / 0.22 lbs cooked green beans
- 1 teaspoon salt
- 1teaspoon black pepper
- 3 tablespoon flour
- 1 teaspoon oregano
- 1 teaspoon rosemary
- 2 teaspoon lemon juice
- 4 teaspoon olive oil

**Directions:**
1. You should take tender lentils for this dish. Otherwise, you will not make

good shape cutlets. Peel the onion and carrot. Then chop it into the small pieces and transfer them together to the blender. Blend it till you get homogenous mass. It is very important to blend the vegetables together – each vegetable will absorb juice from each other. Then sprinkle the mass with salt, black pepper, oregano, rosemary and lemon juice. Continue to blend it for 2 minutes more. Then remove the mass from the blender and transfer the lentils to the blender. Blend it for 1 minute and combine the mass with the vegetable mixture. Stir it carefully. Make the same procedure with the cooked green beans. Then add flour to the mass and stir it carefully. Preheat, the air fryer to 180 C / 360 F. Pour the olive oil into the machine. Make the balls from the lentils mass and press it little. Put the cutlets in the air fryer and cook it for 13 minutes. Serve the dish immediately. Enjoy!

### 271. Simple Roasted Zucchini

Servings:4
Cooking Time: 14 Minutes Roast: 392°f
**Ingredients:**
- Cooking oil spray (sunflower, safflower, or refined coconut)
- 2 zucchini, sliced in ¼- to ½-inch-thick rounds (about 2 cups)
- ¼ teaspoon garlic granules
- ⅛ teaspoon sea salt
- Freshly ground black pepper (optional)

**Directions:**
1. Spray the air fryer basket with oil. Place the zucchini rounds in the basket and spread them out as much as you can. Sprinkle the tops evenly with the garlic, salt, and pepper, if using. Spray with the oil and roast for 7 minutes.
2. Remove the basket from the air fryer, toss or flip the zucchini with a spatula to cook evenly, and spray with oil again. Roast an additional 7 minutes, or until the zucchini rounds are nicely browned and tender.

### 272. Savory Cauliflower Stir-fry

Servings: 4
Cooking Time: 25 Minutes.

**Ingredients:**
- 1 medium-sized head cauliflower cut into florets
- 2 large white onions, thinly sliced
- 5 cloves garlic, minced
- 1 1/2 tablespoons tamari or gluten free tamari
- 1 tablespoon rice vinegar
- 1/2 teaspoon coconut sugar
- 1 tablespoon Sriracha or other favorite hot sauce
- 2 scallions for garnish

**Directions:**
1. Preheat the air fryer to 360F. Place cauliflower florets to the fryer and cook for 10 minutes. If your air fryer is one that has holes in the bottom you'll need to use an air fryer insert.
2. Open the air fryer, shake well the cauliflower and slide back in the compartment.
3. Add the sliced onion, stir and cook 10 more minutes, stirring occasionally.
4. Add garlic, stir and cook 5 more minutes.
5. In a small mixing bowl combine soy sauce, rice vinegar, coconut sugar, Sriracha, salt & pepper.
6. Add the mixture to cauliflower and stir. Cook 5 more minutes. The insert keeps all of the juices inside.
7. To serve sprinkle sliced scallions over the top for garnish.

### 273. Vegan Air Fryer Chips

Servings: 3
Cooking Time: 7-10 Minutes
**Ingredients:**
- 3 large apples, such as Honey crisp, Fuji, Jazz
- 3/4 teaspoon ground cinnamon
- A pinch of salt

**Directions:**
1. Wash apples and then dry them with paper towels.
2. You can core apples or leave seeds inside - its on your preference
3. Preheat the air fryer at 390 degrees F.
4. Using knife, cut the apple sideways into 1/8th inch rounds.
5. In a mixing bowl combine cinnamon and salt.

6. Arrange apples in a single layer and sprinkle or rub some cinnamon and salt mixture.
7. Place apples in a single layer in the air fryer.
8. Cook for 8 minutes, flipping sides half way through.

### 274. Crumble With Blueberry And Custard Compote

Servings: 6
Cooking Time: 30 Minutes
**Ingredients:**
- For the apple filling:
- 1 tablespoon water
- 1 teaspoon cinnamon
- 5 tablespoons brown sugar
- 5 tablespoons raisins, optional
- 8 large apples (around 200 to 220 grams each), peeled and then sliced into not too thin pieces
- Cornstarch solution (2 1/2 teaspoons water mixed with 1 teaspoon cornstarch)
- For the crumble topping:
- 100 grams cold butter, cubed
- 120 grams caster sugar
- 180 grams plain flour
- For the blueberry compote:
- 1 tablespoon caster sugar
- 1 tablespoon lemon juice, optional
- 250 grams fresh blueberries
- For the custard:
- 570 milliliters milk
- 2 tablespoons custard powder
- 1 1/2 tablespoons caster sugar

**Directions:**
1. Preheat the air fryer to 160C.
2. For the apple filling:
3. Except for the cornstarch solution, put the rest of ingredients into a large-sized pan and stir to combine. Cover the pan, turn the heat to medium heat and cook for around 10 minutes or till the apples are softened. Add the cornstarch solution and turn the flame off when the mixture turns slightly thick. Pour into a glass baking dish that will fit your air fryer basket.
4. For the crumble topping:
5. Put the sugar and flour in a mixing bowl or a large-sized bowl and, using a whisk

or fork, mix to combine. Using your fingertips, rub the cubed butter into the flour mixture until it resembles breadcrumbs. Spoon the crumble topping over the filling. Put the baking dish in the air fryer basket and set the timer for 30 minutes or until the topping is slightly brown and crisp.
6. For the blueberry compote:
7. While the crumble is baking, put the ingredients into a small-sized pot and mix to combine. Turn the heat to low heat and cook for about 5 minutes or till the blueberries burst slightly and the compote begins coming together. Set aside.
8. For the custard:
9. Prepare the custard following the custard directions.
10. To assemble:
11. When the apple crumble is cooked, spoon a portion into a serving bowl, top with warm custard, and then spoon 1 tablespoon blueberry compote on the top. Serve!

### 275. Vegan French Fries

Servings: 3
Cooking Time: 25 Minutes
**Ingredients:**
- 1 pound Russet potatoes, peeled and rinced
- 1 tbsp soy sauce
- 1 tbsp flour
- 1 tsp garlic powder
- 1 tsp onion powder
- 1 tsp paprika
- 1 tsp chili powder
- A pinch of black pepper to taste

**Directions:**
1. Slice peeled potatoes into 1/2" French fry strips. You can use a Mandoline Slicer with the julienne blade.
2. Place fries into a large ziplock baggie and add soy sauce. Shake well to distribute.
3. Add flour and seasoning to bag and shake to distribute.
4. Preheat the air fryer to 390 F. Load the appliance with potatoes and cook for 20-25 minutes, depending on potato thickness. Shake couple times during cooking.

5. Serve with dipping sauce you prefer.

### 276. Vegan Air Fryer Green Beans

Servings: 4
Cooking Time: 8 Minutes
**Ingredients:**
- 1 pound Organic Green Beans
- Vegetable oil enough to coat your beans
- 1 tsp sea salt
- Crushed red pepper flanks to taste

**Directions:**
1. Rinse Green Beans well in strainer, dry well. Trim the ends off beans with a kitchen scissors.
2. Spread green beans out on cutting board and spray with oil to coat.
3. Transfer beans to a large mixing bowl, add salt and stir to combine well. Add a little red pepper flakes here because we like them extra spicy.
4. Preheat the air fryer to 390 F. Transfer beans in air fryer basket in a single layer. Cook for 8 minutes. Shake the basket once during cooking. Cook until beans are well done and crispy.

### 277. Amazing Air Fryer Beet Chips

Servings: 3
Cooking Time: 25 Minutes
**Ingredients:**
- 1 pound beet, sliced
- 3 tbsp olive oil
- Sea salt to taste

**Directions:**
1. Slice beets with a mandolin or knife (not too thick!)
2. If using frozen beets, place in a colander and run under warm water until thawed
3. Spread beets on baking sheet, dry them well, then spray with olive oil and sprinkle with sea salt. Stir to combine well.
4. Preheat the air fryer to 350 F. Transfer sliced beet to the frying basket. Cook in Air Fryer for 20 minutes shaking the basket every 5 minutes. Cook until ready and crispy.

### 278. Addictive Zucchini Sticks

Servings:4
Cooking Time: 14 Minutes Fry: 392°f
**Ingredients:**
- 2 small zucchini (about ½ pound)
- ½ teaspoon garlic granules
- ¼ teaspoon sea salt
- ⅛ teaspoon freshly ground black pepper
- 2 teaspoons arrowroot (or cornstarch)
- 3 tablespoons chickpea flour
- 1 tablespoon water
- Cooking oil spray (sunflower, safflower, or refined coconut)

**Directions:**
1. Trim the ends off the zucchini and then cut into sticks about 2 inches long and ½ inch wide. You should end up with about 2 cups of sticks.
2. In a medium bowl, combine the zucchini sticks with the garlic, salt, pepper, arrowroot, and flour. Stir well. Add the water and stir again, using a rubber spatula if you have one.
3. Spray the air fryer basket with oil and add the zucchini sticks, spreading them out as much as possible. Spray the zucchini with oil. Fry for 7 minutes.
4. Remove the basket, gently stir or shake so the zucchini cooks evenly, and spray again with oil. Cook for another 7 minutes, or until tender, nicely browned, and crisp on the outside. Enjoy the sticks plain or with your preferred dipping sauce.

### 279. Cilantro Chutney

Servings:3
Cooking Time: 10 Minutes
**Ingredients:**
- 1 cup fresh cilantro
- ⅓ cup finely shredded unsweetened coconut
- 2 tablespoons chopped fresh ginger
- 3 medium garlic cloves, peeled
- ½ jalapeño, seeds removed
- 1 teaspoon cumin seeds
- ½ teaspoon sea salt
- 2 tablespoons fresh lime juice
- ½ cup water

**Directions:**
1. In a food processor or blender, place the cilantro, coconut, ginger, garlic, and jalapeño. Blend thoroughly, although the mixture shouldn't be totally smooth.

2. Add the cumin, salt, lime juice, and water and blend until thoroughly combined, but with a tiny bit of texture still remaining. Serve cold or at room temperature. This will keep in the fridge for 1 or 2 weeks when stored in an airtight container.

### 280. Delicious Chickpeas Snack

Servings: 4
Cooking Time: 10 Minutes
**Ingredients:**
- 1 15-ounce can chickpeas, drained but not rinsed
- 2 tbsp olive oil
- 1 tsp salt
- 2 tbsp lemon juice

**Directions:**
1. Preheat the Air Fryer to 400F.
2. Combine all ingredients in a mixing bowl and place inside the Air Fryer basket.
3. Cook for 15 minutes until the chickpeas are crisp.

### 281. Cheesy French Fries With Shallots

Servings:3
Cooking Time: 19 Minutes Fry: 392°f
**Ingredients:**
- Cooking oil spray (sunflower, safflower, or refined coconut)
- 1 large potato (russet or Yukon Gold), cut into ¼-inch-thick slices
- 1 teaspoon neutral-flavored oil (sunflower, safflower, or refined coconut)
- ¼ teaspoon sea salt
- ⅛ teaspoon freshly ground black pepper
- 1 large shallot, thinly sliced
- ½ cup plus 2 tablespoons prepared Cheesy Sauce
- 2 tablespoons minced chives or scallions (optional)

**Directions:**
1. Spray the air fryer basket with oil. Set aside.
2. In a medium bowl, toss the potato slices with the oil, salt, and pepper. Place in the air fryer basket and fry for 6 minutes. Remove the air fryer basket, stir or shake (so that the slices cook evenly), and fry for another 4 minutes.
3. Remove. Add the shallots, stir (or shake) again, and fry for another 5 minutes.
4. Make the Cheesy Sauce according to the directions here. Set aside, or keep warm on a very low heat burner.
5. Remove the air fryer basket, stir or shake, and fry for a final 4 minutes, or until the fries and shallots are crisp and browned. Serve topped with Cheesy Sauce—and a sprinkle of chives or scallions if it makes you happy.

### 282. Berbere-spiced Fries

Servings:2
Cooking Time: 20 Minutes Fry: 392°f
**Ingredients:**
- 1 large (about ¾ pound) potato (preferably Yukon Gold, but any kind will do)
- Cooking oil spray (sunflower, safflower, or refined coconut)
- 1 tablespoon neutral-flavored cooking oil (sunflower, safflower, or refined coconut)
- 1 teaspoon coconut sugar
- 1 teaspoon garlic granules
- ½ teaspoon berbere
- ½ teaspoon sea salt
- ¼ teaspoon turmeric
- ¼ teaspoon paprika

**Directions:**
1. Scrub the potato and cut it into French fry shapes (about ¼-inch thick), in relatively uniform pieces. Spray the air fryer basket with oil and set aside.
2. In a medium bowl, toss the potato pieces with the oil, sugar, garlic, berbere, salt, turmeric, and paprika and stir very well (I use a rubber spatula). Place in the air fryer basket and fry for 8 minutes.
3. Remove the air fryer basket and shake (or gently stir) well. Fry for another 8 minutes.
4. Remove one last time, stir or shake, and fry for another 3 to 5 minutes, or until tender and nicely browned. Enjoy while still hot or warm.

### 283. Baked Cherry Pudding

Servings: 4

Cooking Time: 40 Minutes
**Ingredients:**
- 200 g / 0.44 lbs cherry
- 100 g / 0.4 cup water
- 200 g / 0.8 cup almond milk
- 50 g / 0.2 cup soy milk
- 50 g / 1.76 oz starch
- 100 g / 0.22 lbs brown sugar
- 1 teaspoon vanilla sugar
- 40 g / 1.4 oz lemon zest
- 100 g / 0.22 lbs flour

**Directions:**
1. Firstly make the sauce for the pudding. Take the cherries and remove the seeds from it. Transfer them to the blender and blend it for 3 minutes. Then remove the cherry mixture from the blender and transfer it to the big bowl. Sprinkle it with brown sugar and stir it carefully. Then transfer it to the pan and cook it for 10 minutes or till it boiled. Meanwhile, combine flour, starch and vanilla sugar together. Mix it. Add lemon zest and mix it again. Combine soy milk almond milk and water together in the separate bowl. Stir it till you get homogenous mass. Then combine liquid and dry mass together. Mix it with the help of the hand mixer. Preheat, the air fryer to 200 C / 390 F. Pour the pudding into the tray and transfer the tray to the air fryer vessel. Close the lid and cook it for 15 minutes or till you get crunch. Remove the pudding from the tray and pour it with the cherry sauce. Serve it immediately!

### 284. Vegan Portobello Mushroom Pizzas With Hummus

Servings: 4
Cooking Time: 10 Minutes
**Ingredients:**
- 4 large portobello mushrooms
- 1 tbsp balsamic vinegar
- salt and black pepper
- 4 tablespoons oil-free pasta sauce
- 1 clove garlic , minced
- 3 ounces zucchini , shredded, chopped, or julienned (about 1/2 medium)
- 2 tablespoons sweet red pepper , diced
- 4 olives kalamata olives , sliced
- 1 teaspoon dried basil
- 1/2 cups hummus
- Fresh basil leaves or other herbs , minced

**Directions:**
1. Wash mushrooms well. Cut off the stems and remove the gills with a spoon. Pat the insides dry and brush or spray both sides with balsamic vinegar. Sprinkle the inside with salt and pepper.
2. Spread 1 tablespoon of pasta sauce inside each mushroom and sprinkle it with garlic.
3. Preheat the Air Fryer to 330F.
4. Place as many mushrooms as will fit in a single layer. Cook for 3 minutes.
5. Remove mushrooms and top each one with equal portions of zucchini, peppers, and olives and sprinkle with dried basil and salt and pepper.
6. Return to the Air Fryer and cook for another 3 minutes or more until mushrooms are tender.
7. When ready transfer to the plate, drizzle with hummus and sprinkle with basil or other herbs.

### 285. Onion Pie

Servings: 4
Cooking Time: 45 Minutes
**Ingredients:**
- 150 g / 0.33 lbs flour
- 50 g / 0.2 cup almond milk
- 1 teaspoon salt
- 50 g / 0.2 cup water
- 300 g / 0.66 lbs onion
- 1 teaspoon olive oil
- 100 g / 0.22 lbs tofu
- 50 g / 0.2 cup soy milk
- 4 tomatoes

**Directions:**
1. Peel the onion and chop it into the small pieces. Transfer the chopped onion to the big mixing bowl and sprinkle it with salt. Then chop the tofu cheese and add it to the mixing bowl too. Stir it gently till you get homogenous mass. Take small tomatoes for this dish and cut it into two parts. Then leave the mixture with chopped onion and take another bowl and sift flour in it. Add soy milk

and almond milk. Take the hand mixture and mix the mass very carefully. Preheat the air fryer to 200 C / 390 F. Meanwhile, take the pie tray and spray it with olive oil. Knead dough very carefully. Then put it on the tray and make it flat. Transfer the onion mixture on the dough and add tomato halves. Take another vessel and pour water in it. Transfer the vessel with water to the air fryer and put the tray with pie in it. Close the lid and reduce the temperature to 180 C / 360 F and cook the pie for 20 minutes. Then open the lid and leave it for 10 minutes more. Enjoy!

### 286. Vegan Falafel

Servings: 8
Cooking Time: 15 Minutes
**Ingredients:**
- 1 ½ cups dry garbanzo beans
- ½ cup chopped fresh parsley
- ½ cup chopped fresh cilantro
- ½ cup chopped white onion
- 7 cloves garlic, minced
- 2 tbsp all purpose flour
- A pinch of salt
- 1 tbsp ground cumin
- ⅛ tsp ground cardamom
- 1 tsp ground coriander
- ⅛ tsp cayenne pepper

**Directions:**
1. Place dried garbanzo beans in a large bowl and cover with 1 inch of water. Soak overnight. Drain thoroughly.
2. In a food processor bowl add parsley, cilantro, onion and garlic. Mix until well combined.
3. Add soaked garbanzo beans, flour, salt, cumin, cardamom, coriander and cayenne to food processor. Pulse until ingredients form a rough, coarse meal. Scrape down sides of food processor occasionally.
4. Transfer mixture to a bowl, cover and cool in fridge for 1-2 hours.
5. After that form 1 inch balls and flatten them to form patties.
6. Preheat the air fryer to 390 F. Lightly spray fryer basket with oil if desired. Place falafel into basket in one layer.

Cook for 10 minutes, turning halfway through. Repeat with remaining falafel.
7. Serve.

### 287. Sesame Crunch Tofu

Servings:3
Cooking Time: 20 Minutes Bake: 392°f
**Ingredients:**
- 1 (8-ounce) package tofu, firm or extra-firm
- 1½ tablespoons tamari or shoyu
- ½ teaspoon granulated garlic
- ⅓ cup sesame seeds (raw, untoasted)
- 2 teaspoons flour (whole-wheat pastry, chickpea, or brown rice)
- 1 tablespoon arrowroot (or cornstarch)
- 2 tablespoons neutral-flavored oil (sunflower, safflower, or refined coconut)
- Cooking oil spray (sunflower, safflower, or refined coconut)

**Directions:**
1. Slice the tofu into ½-inch thick slabs, and then into triangles.
2. Press the tofu by placing the pieces in a single file layer on top of paper towels (or a tea towel) then covering with additional towel(s). Press down gently, yet firmly, to remove any excess moisture.
3. Place the pressed tofu on a plate. Sprinkle evenly with the tamari and garlic. Turn to coat well.
4. In a medium bowl, combine the sesame seeds, flour, and arrowroot. Add the tofu and stir well, yet gently, with a rubber spatula so the pieces are evenly coated with the sesame mixture. Add the oil, and stir one last time to coat the tofu.
5. Spray your air fryer basket with oil. Place the tofu in a single layer in your air fryer basket and bake for 10 minutes. Remove. Turn the pieces over and cook for another 10 minutes, or until golden-brown and crisp. Remove and enjoy.

### 288. Festive Vegetable Stew

Servings: 4
Cooking Time: 40 Minutes
**Ingredients:**
- 300 g / 0.66 lbs tomatoes

- 200 g / 0.44 lbs zucchini
- 1 onion
- 2 green sweet peppers
- 1 yellow sweet pepper
- 100 g / 0.22 lbs tomato paste
- 100 g / 0.4 cup almond milk
- 1 teaspoon cilantro
- 1 teaspoon chili pepper
- 100 g / 0.22 lbs leek
- 100 g / 0.22 lbs lentils
- 300 g / 1.2 cup vegetables stock

**Directions:**
1. Chop the tomatoes on the very small pieces. Then slice the zucchini and cut it into two parts more. Remove the seeds from the sweet pepper and cut it into the strips. Then cut each strip into two parts more. Chop the leek. Take the big bowl and combine all ingredients together in it. Stir it gently. Then add lentils to it and sprinkle the mass with the cilantro, chili pepper, and tomato paste. Stir it carefully and leave it. Preheat the air fryer to 200 C / 390 F. Meanwhile, peel the onion and chop it roughly. Combine vegetable stock with almond milk together and stir it. Then pour the liquid into the air fryer and add vegetable mass. Stir it gently with the help of the wooden spoon. Close the lid and cook it for 20 minutes. The lentils should absorb all water. Then remove the stew, chill it little and serve it immediately.

### 289. Air Fryer Jicama Fries Recipe

Servings: 2
Cooking Time: 15 Minutes
**Ingredients:**
- 1 large Jicama, cut into matchsticks
- ½ tsp of garlic powder
- 1 tsp of smoked paprika
- 2 tbsp olive or sesame oil
- A pinch of salt and pepper to taste

**Directions:**
1. In a large mixing bowl, add the jicama matchsticks. Sprinkle with olive oil and season with garlic powder, smoked paprika, salt and pepper. Stir to combine well.
2. Preheat the air fryer to 390 F. Fry for about 12-15 minutes depending on

quantity and shake 2-3 times during cooking. Cook until brown and crispy.
3. Serve hot with ketchup or your favorite dipping sauce.

### 290. Leek Cutlets

Servings: 4
Cooking Time: 30 Minutes
**Ingredients:**
- 300 g / 0.66 lbs leek
- 1 teaspoon salt
- 200 g / 0.44 lbs onion
- 1 teaspoon olive oil
- 1 teaspoon oregano
- 1 teaspoon basil
- 1 teaspoon chili pepper
- 1 tablespoon flour
- 1 carrot

**Directions:**
1. Chop the leek and transfer it to the big mixing bowl. Then sprinkle it with chili pepper, basil, oregano, and salt. Stir it carefully. Peel the onion and cut it into 6 parts. Transfer the onion to the blender and blend it till you get a smooth mixture. Then transfer the onion mass to the mixing bowl with the chopped leek. Peel the carrot and grate it. Add the grated carrot into the mixing bowl too. Stir the mixture very carefully. If it is dry, enough you can knead it as a dough. Preheat the air fryer to 180 C / 360 F and spray the air fryer vessel with olive oil. Then make the cutlets from the vegetable mixture and sprinkle the cutlets with the flour. Transfer the vegetable "balls" to the air fryer and close the lid. Cook it for 12 minutes. Serve it immediately. Enjoy!

### 291. Vegan Maple Cinnamon Buns

Servings: 4
Cooking Time: 30 Minutes
**Ingredients:**
- 3/4 cup unsweetened almond milk
- 4 tbsp maple syrup
- 1 ½ tbsp active yeast
- 1 tbsp ground flaxseed
- 1 tbsp coconut oil, melted
- 1 cup wholegrain flour, sifted
- 1 ½ cup plain white flour, sifted
- 2 tsp cinnamon

- ½ cup pecan nuts, toasted
- 2 ripe bananas, sliced
- 4 Medjool dates, pitted
- ¼ cup icing sugar

**Directions:**
1. Heat the ¾ cup almond milk to lukewarm and add the maple syrup and yeast. Allow the yeast to activate for 5 to 10 minutes.
2. Meanwhile, in a large mixing bowl combine flaxseed and 3 tablespoons of water to make the egg replacement. Allow flaxseed to soak for 2 minutes.
3. Add the coconut oil. Pour the flaxseed mixture to the yeast mixture. Mix well.
4. In another bowl, combine two types of flour and the 1 tablespoon cinnamon powder.
5. Pour the yeast-flaxseed mixture and combine until dough forms.
6. Knead the dough on a floured surface for at least 10 minutes.
7. Place the kneaded dough in a greased bowl and cover with a kitchen towel. Leave in a warm and dark area for the bread to rise for 1 hour.
8. Meanwhile, in a bowl combine pecans, banana slices, and dates. Add 1 tablespoon of cinnamon powder. Stir to combine.
9. Preheat the air fryer to 390F. Roll the risen dough on a floured surface until it is thin. Spread the pecan mixture on to the dough.
10. Roll the dough and cut into nine slices. Transfer to the air fryer basket and cook for about 25-30 minutes.
11. Once cooked, sprinkle with icing sugar and serve.

### 292. Air Fryer Sweet Potato Hash Browns

Servings: 4
Cooking Time: 20 Minutes
**Ingredients:**
- 4 medium-sized sweet potatoes, peeled
- 2 garlic cloves, minced
- 1 tsp cinnamon
- 1 tsp paprika
- Salt and pepper, to taste
- 2 tbsp olive oil

**Directions:**
1. Grate the sweet potatoes using the largest holes of a cheese grater.
2. Soak grated sweet potatoes in a bowl of cold water for 20 minutes. Soaking the sweet potatoes in cold water will help remove the starch from the potatoes. This makes them crunchy.
3. Drain the water from the potatoes and dry them completely using a paper towel.
4. Place the potatoes in a dry bowl. Add the olive oil, garlic, paprika, and salt and pepper to taste. Stir to combine the ingredients.
5. Preheat the air fryer to 370 F. Add the potatoes to the air fryer and cook for 15-20 minutes shaking couple times during cooking.
6. Cool before serving.

### 293. Whole Wheat Eggless Chocolate Chips Cookies

Servings: 6
Cooking Time: 10 Minutes
**Ingredients:**
- 1 cup whole-wheat flour
- 1/2-3/4 cup powdered sugar or castor sugar
- 1/2 cup unsalted vegan butter (I used I Can't Believe It's Not Butter)
- 1/4 baking powder
- 2 teaspoons nut milk
- 2 teaspoons vegan chocolate chips (I used Enjoy Life)

**Directions:**
1. Put the baking powder, flour, and butter in a mixing bowl. With your fingers, rub the ingredients together until the mixture resembles breadcrumbs.
2. Add the milk, sugar, and chocolate chips. Mix to incorporate – the dough should be soft but firm. Refrigerate 15 to 20 minutes.
3. When the dough is firm, form into balls and then flatten into cookie shapes. If desired, you can use a cookie cutter to shape them. Glaze the top of the cookies with a bit of milk.
4. Put the cookie doughs into a preheated 160C air fryer for 10 minutes. Set the timer for 10 minutes cooking.

5. When the timer beeps, let it sit in on standby mode for 10 minutes, allowing the cookies to cool inside the air fryer.
6. Store leftovers in an airtight container.

### 294. Air Fried Cauliflower Rice

Servings: 3
Cooking Time: 20 Minutes
**Ingredients:**
- Round 1
- 1/2 block firm or extra firm tofu
- 2 tbsp low sodium soy sauce
- 1 medium-sized onion, diced
- 1 medium carrot, diced
- 1 tsp turmeric
- Round 2
- 3 cups riced cauliflower - Cauliflower minced into pieces smaller than the size of a pea. You can do this by hand with a box-style cheese crater, use your food processor to pulse into pieces, or buy pre-riced, bagged cauliflower.
- 2 tbsp low sodium soy sauce
- 1 tbsp sesame oil
- 1 tbsp rice vinegar
- 1 tbsp minced ginger
- 1/2 cup finely chopped broccoli
- 2 cloves garlic, minced
- 1/2 cup frozen peas

**Directions:**
1. In a large bowl, crumble the tofu, then toss with the rest of the Round 1 ingredients.
2. Preheat the air fryer to 370 F and cook for about 8-10 minutes, shaking once.
3. Meanwhile, in another mixing bowl toss together all of the Round 2 ingredients.
4. When that first 10 minutes of cooking are done, add all of the Round 2 ingredients to your air fryer, shake gently, and fry at 370 for 10 more minutes, shaking after 5 minutes.
5. Cook until ready and brown.
6. Serve and enjoy.

### 295. Fruit Pudding

Servings: 4
Cooking Time: 35 Minutes
**Ingredients:**
- 100 g / 0.22 lbs strawberry
- 50 g / 1.76 oz pineapple
- 1 peach
- 1 teaspoon vanilla sugar
- 50 g / 1.76 oz sugar
- 100 g / 0.4 cup almond milk
- 50 g / 0.2 cup coconut milk
- 2 teaspoon water
- 70 g / 2.5 oz starch
- 1 teaspoon honey
- 50 g / 1.76 oz flour

**Directions:**
1. Take the big bowl and combine cocoa milk, almond milk and vanilla sugar together. Then add starch and water. Stir it gently and add flour. Take the hand mixer and mix it till you get homogenous mass. Preheat the air fryer to 200 C / 390 F. Take the fruits and wash it. Then slice it roughly. Take the pudding and pour it into the pudding tray and transfer the tray to the air fryer vessel. Then add sliced fruits and close the lid. Cook it for 15 minutes. Look at the fruits – they will make you understand that the pudding is ready because of crunch. Then open the lid and leave it for 10 minutes more. Pour the cooked pudding with honey and serve it immediately!

### 296. Air Fryer Vegan Garlic Mushrooms

Servings: 2
Cooking Time: 15 Minutes
**Ingredients:**
- 1/2 pound mushrooms
- 1 tbsp olive or sesame oil
- 1/2 tsp garlic powder
- 1 tsp Worcestershire or soy sauce
- A pinch of kosher salt , to taste
- Freshly ground black pepper , to taste
- Lemon wedges (optional)
- 1 tbsp chopped parsley

**Directions:**
1. Wash and dry mushrooms. Cut mushrooms in half or quarters (depending on preferred size).
2. In a large mixing bowl add mushrooms and toss with oil, garlic powder, Worcestershire/soy sauce, salt and pepper. Stir to combine.
3. Preheat the air fryer to 375 F. Cook mushrooms for about 10-12 minutes, shaking couple times half way through.

4. Squeeze lemon and top with chopped parsley.

### 297. Fragrant Quinoa

Servings: 4
Cooking Time: 30 Minutes
**Ingredients:**
- 200 g / 0.44 lbs quinoa
- 300 g / 1.2 cup vegetable stock
- 1 teaspoon chili pepper
- 1 teaspoon rosemary
- 1 teaspoon basil
- 1 teaspoon turmeric
- 1 teaspoon cilantro
- 100 g / 0.4 cup spinach
- 10 g / 0.35 oz fresh mint
- 200 g / 0.44 lbs tomatoes
- 1 red sweet pepper
- 1 teaspoon black pepper

**Directions:**
1. Take the small bowl and combine chili pepper, rosemary, basil, turmeric, cilantro, and spinach. Stir the mixture very carefully. Then remove the seeds from the sweet pepper and chop it. Sprinkle the chopped peppers with the black pepper and stir it gently. Chop the tomatoes and mint. Take the big bowl and transfer all ingredients in it then sprinkle the mass with the spice mixture and stir it carefully. Leave it. Meanwhile, preheat the air fryer to 200 C / 390 F. Transfer the mixture to the air fryer and pour it with vegetable stock. Mix it with the help of a wooden spoon. Close the lid and reduce the heat of the air fryer to 180 C / 360 F. Cook the quinoa for 15 minutes or till it absorbs all water. Close the lid and remove the dish from the air fryer. Serve it immediately.

### 298. Delicious Cutlets

Servings: 4
Cooking Time: 30 Minutes
**Ingredients:**
- 200 g / 0.44 lbs onion
- 1 carrot
- 2 teaspoon flour
- 1 teaspoon soy milk
- 10 g / 0.35 oz tofu
- 1 teaspoon olive oil
- 1 teaspoon black pepper
- 1teaspoon salt
- 1 egg

**Directions:**
1. The main secret of every type of the vegetable cutlet is in the size of ingredients. Peel the onion and carrot. Then chop the onion on the very small pieces. You can even use a blender for this procedure. Then remove the juice from the onion and transfer the mass to the big bowl. Grate the carrot. You should make it very thick and combine the vegetable with the chopped onion. Stir it and sprinkle the mass with the black pepper, salt, and flour. Stir it. Then whisk the egg. Combine it with the teaspoon of soy milk. Grate the tofu and add it to the egg mixture. Stir it again. Preheat, the air fryer to the 180 C / 360 F. Make the balls from the vegetable mixture. Then press every ball little and transfer them to the preheated air fryer. Pour the balls with eggs mixture and close the lid. Cook it for 15 minutes and serve it immediately.

### 299. Air Fryer Spicy Tofu

Servings: 2
Cooking Time: 20 Minutes
**Ingredients:**
- 1 package tofu
- 1/2 cup plain flour
- Chopped green onion for garnish
- Sesame seeds
- 1 tsp sesame or avocado oil
- For garlic sauce
- 4 tbsp liquid aminos
- 1 tbsp rice vinegar
- 1 tbsp chili sauce
- 1 tbsp agave nectar
- 2 garlic cloves, minced
- 1 tbsp ginger, grated

**Directions:**
1. Cut the tofu into cubes.
2. In a large sealable bag, toss the tofu and flour vigorously until all of the tofu is coated.
3. Preheat the air fryer to 360 F. Working in batches, place the tofu into the air fryer leaving enough space between the pieces and sprinkle lightly with oil.

4. Cook for 20 minutes shaking once while cooking. Fry until crisp.
5. Meanwhile, prepare the ginger garlic sauce. Place all of the ingredients into a large mixing bowl and whisk until well combined.
6. After all of the tofu is crispy, transfer it to frying pan. Over medium heat, pour the sauce over the crispy tofu and stir to coat. Allow the tofu and sauce to heat until the sauce has reduced by half. About 3 minutes.
7. Serve over rice or with toothpicks for a fun appetizer.
8. Enjoy!

## 300. Classic French Fries

Servings:3
Cooking Time: 22 Minutes Fry: 392°f
**Ingredients:**
- 2 medium potatoes, preferably Yukon Gold (but any kind will do)
- Cooking oil spray (sunflower, safflower, or refined coconut)
- 2 teaspoons oil (olive, sunflower, or melted coconut)
- ½ teaspoon garlic granules
- ¼ teaspoon plus ⅛ teaspoon sea salt
- ¼ teaspoon freshly ground black pepper
- ¼ teaspoon paprika
- Ketchup, hot sauce, or No-Dairy Ranch Dressing, for serving

**Directions:**
1. Scrub the potatoes and cut them into French fry shapes (about ¼-inch thick), in relatively uniform sizes. Spray the air fryer basket with oil and set aside.
2. In a medium bowl, toss the cut potato pieces with the oil, garlic, salt, pepper, and paprika and stir very well (I use a rubber spatula). Place in an air fryer basket and fry for 8 minutes.
3. Remove the air fryer basket and shake (or gently stir) well. Fry for another 8 minutes. Remove one last time, stir or shake, and fry for another 6 minutes, or until tender and nicely browned. Enjoy plain or with ketchup, hot sauce, vegan ranch, or any other sauce that flips your fancy.

## 301. Savory Cauliflower Chickpea Tacos

Servings: 4
Cooking Time: 20 Minutes
**Ingredients:**
- 4 cups cauliflower florets cut into bite-sized pieces
- 1 can of chickpeas drained and rinsed
- 2 tablespoons olive oil
- 2 tablespoons taco seasoning
- To serve
- 8 small tortillas
- 2 middle-sized avocados sliced
- 4 cups cabbage shredded
- Coconut yogurt to drizzle

**Directions:**
1. In a large mixing bowl mix cauliflower florets and chickpeas with the olive oil and taco seasoning.
2. Preheat the air fryer to 390 F.
3. Transfer the mixture to the air fryer basket and cook for about 18-20 minutes, stirring occasionally until cooked. Please be noticed that cauliflower will be golden but not burnt.
4. Serve in tacos with avocado slices, cabbage and coconut yogurt and enjoy!

## 302. Kiwi Pudding

Servings: 4
Cooking Time: 45 Minutes
**Ingredients:**
- 100 g / 0.22 lbs kiwi
- 200 g / 0.8 cup orange juice
- 1 teaspoon vanilla sugar
- 50 g / 1.76 oz brown sugar
- 60 g / 2.1 oz starch
- 1 teaspoon lemon juice
- 20 g / 0.7 oz lemon zest
- 50 g / 0.2 cup almond milk
- 4 teaspoon flour

**Directions:**
1. Slice the kiwi on the small pieces. Then combine the orange juice with almond milk and lemon juice. Mix it gently. Take the big bowl and combine sugar, vanilla sugar, lemon zest and flour together. Stir it very carefully and add starch. Then combine liquid and dry mixtures together and pour it into the pan. Cook it on the medium heat for 5 minutes. Till you get thick mass.

Meanwhile, preheat the air fryer to 200 C / 390 F. Remove the pudding from the oven and transfer it to the tray then put the tray in the air fryer and add sliced kiwi. Stir the mass very gently with the help of the wooden spoon. Close the lid and cook it for 20 minutes. Then leave the pudding for 10 minutes more and serve it immediately. Enjoy!

### 303. Cabbage Cutlets

Servings: 4
Cooking Time: 30 Minutes
**Ingredients:**
- 200 g / 0.44 lbs cabbage
- 100 g / 0.22 lbs kale
- 1 teaspoon salt
- 1teaspoon black pepper
- 1 teaspoon chili pepper
- 50 g / 0.2 cup soy milk
- 100 g / 0.4 cup water
- 1 teaspoon starch
- 1 teaspoon oregano
- 2 tablespoon flour

**Directions:**
1. Grate the cabbage. Take the kale and chop it roughly. Transfer the chopped kale to the blender. Blend it for 4 minutes. Remove the mixture from the blender and combine it with grated cabbage in the big bowl. Sprinkle it with black and chili pepper. Add oregano, starch and flour. Stir it carefully. Add salt and stir it again. Then preheat the air fryer to 180 C / 360 F. Meanwhile make the sauce for cutlets: combine soy milk with water. Mix it. Pour the mass to the air fryer. Make the balls from the cabbage mass. You can press them little or transfer the balls directly to the air fryer vessel. Cook it for 10 minutes. Remove the cutlets from the air fryer and transfer them to the serving plate. Pour the cooked dish with the sauce. Enjoy!

### 304. Spicy Air Fryer Vegetables

Servings: 4
Cooking Time: 35 Minutes
**Ingredients:**
- 4 carrots
- 200 g / 0.44 lbs broccoli
- 3 tomatoes
- 2 white small onions
- 20 g / 0.7 oz rosemary
- 1 teaspoon salt
- 1 teaspoon black pepper
- 1 teaspoon chili pepper
- 1 teaspoon basil
- 2 tablespoon olive oil
- 1 teaspoon cilantro
- 100 g / 0.22 lbs garlic
- 200 g / 0.44 lbs leek

**Directions:**
1. You can chop all the vegetables or do not make the pieces. Take the carrots and wash it. Peel it and cut the vegetable into the thick strips. Make sure that there are no thin strips – otherwise, it will be burnt in the air fryer. Then peel the onion and cut it into the four pieces. Take the big bowl and transfer the vegetables to it. Then mix the onion to make a lot of small pieces. Cut the leek into the strips and make the florets from the broccoli. Transfer the vegetables to the big mixing bowl too. Sprinkle the vegetable mixture with rosemary, salt, black pepper, chili pepper, basil, and cilantro. Stir it carefully. Then crush the garlic with skin and add it to the vegetables. Chop the tomatoes and put them directly in the air fryer. Add vegetable mass and stir it gently with the help of a wooden spoon. Then spray the vegetables with olive oil and close the lid. Cook it in 180 C / 360 F for 20 minutes. Serve it immediately.

### 305. Potato Cutlets

Servings: 5
Cooking Time: 20 Minutes
**Ingredients:**
- 300 g / 0.66 lbs mashed potato
- 1 onion
- 1 carrot
- 2 tablespoon rice flour
- 1 teaspoon black pepper
- 2 teaspoon water
- 1 tablespoon olive oil
- 50 g / 1.76 oz chopped dill

**Directions:**

1. Take the big mixing bowl and transfer the mashed potato in it. Sprinkle it with black pepper and chopped dill. Stir it carefully. Then peel the onion. Chop it. Take the skillet and pour the olive oil. Cook the chopped onion till it browned. Then transfer the onion to the mashed potato. Peel the carrot and grate it. Add grated carrot to the potato mass. Add rice flour and stir it carefully again. Preheat, the air fryer to 180 C / 360 F. Pour the water in the air fryer vessel. Make the cutlets from the potato mixture and transfer them to the preheated air fryer. Cook it for 7 minutes. Serve it immediately.

carefully and leave it. Meanwhile, preheat the air fryer to 200 C / 390 F. Pour water into the air fryer vessel and then transfer all other ingredients and stir it gently. Close the lid and cook it for 15 minutes. Then remove the dish from the air fryer and sprinkle it with the chopped parsley. Serve it immediately.

**306. Delicious Green Beans**

Servings: 3
Cooking Time: 30 Minutes
**Ingredients:**
- 100 g / 0.22 lbs green beans
- 2 sweet green peppers
- 1 teaspoon chili pepper
- 50 g / 1.76 oz asparagus
- 2 teaspoon lemon juice
- 1 teaspoon olive oil
- 1 teaspoon black pepper
- 1teaspoon basil
- 1 teaspoon chopped dill
- 1 teaspoon chopped parsley
- 200 g / 0.8 cup water

**Directions:**
1. It is low fat and delight dish. Make sure that you do not make a very small piece of every ingredient. Wash the green beans and asparagus. Then cut every ingredient into 2 parts and transfer them to the big bowl. Remove the seeds from the green peppers and cut it into 4 parts then cut every part into 2 pieces. Add the pepper's pieces to the bowl with the asparagus and green beans. Stir it very gently to not destroy the ingredients. Sprinkle the mixture with the lemon juice, olive oil, chili pepper, black pepper and chopped dill – take the dried dill for this dish. Stir it

CPSIA information can be obtained
at www.ICGtesting.com
Printed in the USA
BVHW012237311021
620416BV00003B/67